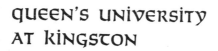

THE COMMON COLD AND THE FLU

The Common Cold and the Flu

BY NATHAN AASENG

Franklin Watts
New York/Chicago/London/Toronto/Sydney
A Venture Book

Photographs copyright © : The Bettmann Archive: p. 13;
Photo Researchers, Inc.: pp. 16 (National Library
of Medicine/SPL), 25, 31 (both Omikron), 28 (M. Wurtz,
Biozentrum/SPL), 29 (Biophoto Associates), 36, 37, 39
(all David M. Phillips/Population Council); North Wind
Picture Archives, Alfred, ME: pp. 18, 20; University of
Wisconsin, Madison/Jay Salvo: p. 33; UPI/Bettmann
Newsphotos: pp. 46, 52; Randy Matusow: pp. 56, 62, 70;
Purdue University News Service: pp. 76 (David Umberger), 77;
Dr. Richard J. Colonno/Bristol-Myers Squibb
Pharmaceutical Research Institute: p. 81.

Library of Congress Cataloging-in-Publication Data

Aaseng, Nathan.
    The common cold and the flu / by Nathan Aaseng,
        p.   cm. — (A Venture book.)
    Includes bibliographical references and index.
    Summary: Discusses the causes, symptoms, methods of prevention,
and treatment of two common ailments, colds and flus.
    ISBN 0-531-12537-8
    1. Influenza—Juvenile liturature.   2. Cold (Disease)—Juvenile
literature.   [1. Influenza.   2. Cold (Disease)]   I. Title.
RC150.A25   1992
616.2′05—dc20   92-15137 CIP AC

CONTENTS

1
What Do You Know About Colds and Flu?
9

2
The Mystery of Colds and Flu
15

3
Viral Wars
27

4
Vaccination: Deception and Counterdeception
44

5
Preventing Colds and Flu: Facts and Fallacies
55

6
Treating Colds and Flu: Facts and Fallacies
66

7
The Future of Colds and Flu
75

Glossary
86

For Further Reading
89

Index
91

THE COMMON COLD
AND THE FLU

1

WHAT DO YOU KNOW ABOUT COLDS AND FLU?

Yesterday Jennifer Allen took her health for granted. This morning she can appreciate what a blessing good health is, because she feels awful. She was fine when she went to bed last night, but sometime after midnight she started shivering and felt her throat go dry. Now she is coughing, she's tired, her nose is running, her forehead could pass for a hot griddle, and her body feels as though it's been used as a punching bag.

"Not you, too!" sighs her mother as Jennifer trudges down the hall, sniffling. "I was afraid of this when I heard you coughing last night. Well, it's no wonder, the way you walk around after a shower with that wet head this time of year in a chilly house! I'm just surprised you don't catch more colds."

"I think this is the worst one I've ever had. Feel my forehead."

"Hmmm," says Mom, touching her warm skin. "I don't like that. Maybe it's not just a *cold*. Could be the *flu*."

"I don't think so. If I had the flu, wouldn't my stomach be upset?" Jennifer says, shaking her head. She coughs again into her fist.

"At any rate, I think you'd better stay home from school today," says Mom.

"No way!" Jennifer wails. "I've got too much to do."

"But you can't go anywhere feeling like this," Mom insists. "Why don't you just take it easy in bed awhile? I'll stay home from work and fix you some hot tea for breakfast and chicken soup for lunch."

"I can't," Jennifer protests. "I've got a math test this morning, and I don't want to fall behind. Besides, we have a basketball game today. If we win, we'll be in first place."

"You're just like your father," Mom sighs, as Dad walks into the room. "I can't get him to slow down either."

"It's just a cold," says Dad, blowing into a handkerchief. Even after his shower he still smelled slightly of that menthol ointment he had rubbed on his chest the night before. "If everybody stayed in bed each time they got a cold, nothing would ever get done. When you have a cold, you just have to tough it out. Here," he says, tossing Jennifer a bottle from the cupboard. "Vitamin C. Take two of these tablets every two hours and you'll stay on top of that cold."

"You and your health fads," says Mom, shaking her head.

"Vitamin C isn't a fad; there's scientific proof it works," says Dad. "And what do you call chicken soup? That's plain, old-fashioned superstition," teases Dad.

"I suppose it won't hurt," coughs Jennifer, as she looks at the vitamin bottle. "But I'd rather take one of those multi-purpose cold medicines to get me through the day. We still have some, don't we?"

"Yes, I think so," says Mom. "But you know what they say about colds. 'A cold treated with the best medicines can be cured in just seven days. Left alone, it could last as long as a week!'"

"I've got to go," says Dad. "Hope you're feeling better tonight, sweetheart." He gives Jennifer a quick kiss and leans down to offer the same to his wife.

"What are you thinking of?" Mom says, as she backs away. "I don't want to catch your cold."

"A kiss wouldn't hurt you," sniffs Dad as he heads out the door. "A person is *contagious* only during the *incubation* time, before all the *symptoms* start. I'm perfectly safe now."

A MOST FAMILIAR ILLNESS

The Allen family is dealing with one of the most familiar health hazards known to humans, the upper respiratory viral infection. The milder form of this infection, known medically as *viral rhinitis,* strikes so often that it has come to be called the common cold. Last year nearly a billion cases of the common cold occurred in the United States alone, more cases than all other diseases combined.

Because a cold is a relatively mild illness, people tend to regard it lightly. A cold is viewed as a nuisance, like a cut finger or skinned knees. You treat it with something in your medicine cabinet and do your best to pretend it's not there until it goes away.

Yet this supposedly innocent infection is a significant drain on our society. The delay of the launching of a space shuttle flight in early 1990 illustrates the mischief that can be caused by a single case of the common cold. The flight had to be postponed a week, primarily because crew commander John Crieghton had come down with a cold and was too sick to fly. The cost of the delay was estimated at more than $2.5 million!

Every year the common cold costs the United States more than 30 million missed days of work or school, making it the leading cause of job and school absences. Although a cold almost always runs its course without needing professional treatment, colds nevertheless prompt· more doctor visits, ($3 billion worth per year in the United States), than any other condition. On top of that, Americans spend $2 billion each year on over-the-counter cold remedies.

Influenza, the upper respiratory infection from which

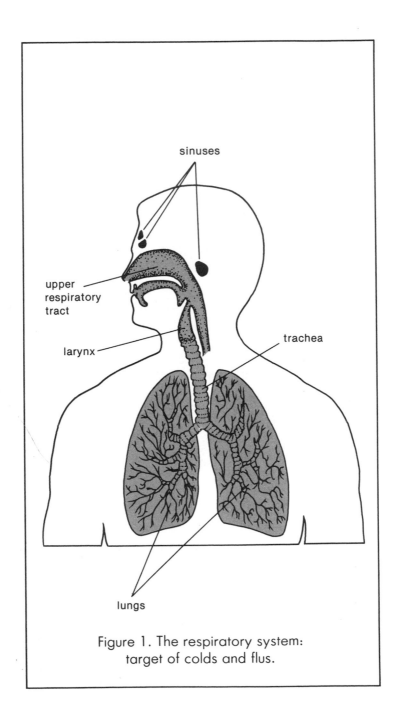

Figure 1. The respiratory system:
target of colds and flus.

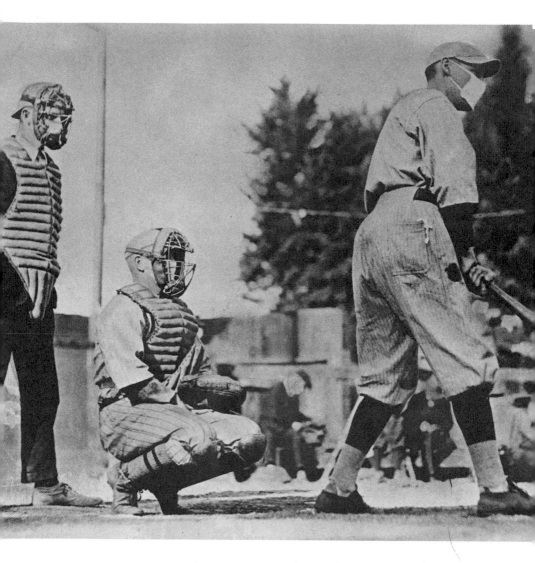

Batter, catcher, umpire, and crowd wear surgical
masks in this photo of a baseball game held
during the 1918–19 influenza pandemic. An
estimated 20 million people died during
this epidemic, which occurred in the
aftermath of World War 1.

Jennifer Allen was actually suffering, brings a number of more serious problems. The flu, short for *influenza,* has been one of the deadliest diseases of the twentieth century. A particularly lethal strain of flu swept the world in 1918–19, infecting about 85 percent of the population of all countries. An estimated 20 million people died of the disease during those years. Since then, major outbreaks of flu have occurred every ten to fifteen years. More than 500,000 deaths have been attributed to the flu in the United States over the past twenty years. Individuals at the highest risk are the elderly, those with chronic respiratory problems, and those with weakened *immune systems.*

Colds and flu visit our homes so frequently that we ought to know them well, and should be well prepared for their attacks. Yet as familiar as these illnesses may be, they remain a source of mystery and confusion. Even the experts cannot totally agree on such basics as what causes colds and flu, how they are spread, and what should be done to treat them.

Like many people, Jennifer Allen and her parents *think* they know a great deal about colds and how to deal with them. How much do they really know? How much do *you* know? Can you pick out the accuracies and the errors in the statements made by the Allen family?

2

THE MYSTERY OF COLDS AND FLU

*H*umans have been sniffling and coughing from colds and flu since the beginning of recorded medical history. As early as 412 B.C., the Greek physician Hippocrates described an *epidemic* of what appears to be influenza. ("Epidemic" refers to a large number of infections in a local population. The word "pandemic" is used to describe widespread infection over a number of countries.)

In ancient times, many theories arose as to what caused upper respiratory illnesses. Some believed that a runny nose was merely nature's way of eliminating waste products from the brain. Others believed that these sicknesses were spread to humans from contact with horses. Still others traced the outbreaks of flu to the position of the planets or to the influence of comets and meteors. The term "influenza" was coined by Italians during a flu epidemic in 1504, and refers to the "influence" of the heavenly bodies. The English adopted the word in the eighteenth century, during one of the 31 pandemics that have occurred since the early 1500s.

One of the earliest prime suspects in the cause of upper respiratory ailments has been the air. For centuries doctors believed that some kind of poisonous gas was dispersed through the air, perhaps let loose by earthquakes

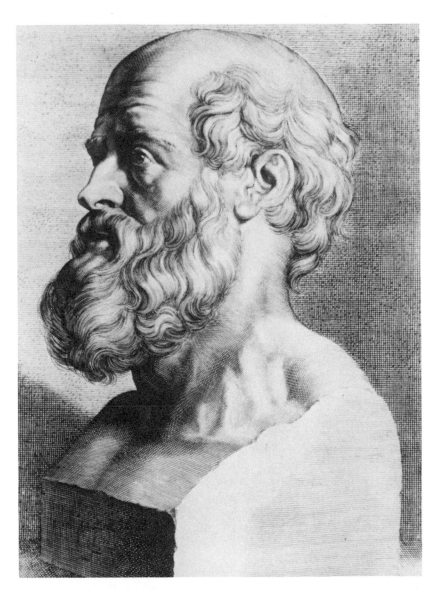

The Greek physician Hippocrates (460–370 B.C), considered the "father of medicine," lived on the Aegean island of Cos. He is believed to have made the first record of an influenza epidemic.

or volcanoes, that produced disease in the breathing passages. As late as the nineteenth century, physicians were still pointing to this foul "*miasma*" as they called it, as the culprit in colds and flu.

Other evidence pointed to the weather as the agent of disease. The common cold got its name from the widespread belief that exposure to cold weather brought about the illness. When George Washington came down with a bad cold on December 12, 1799, the illness was blamed on the fact that he had taken a long horseback ride in subfreezing, snowy weather. Another United States president, William Henry Harrison, died in office of a severe infection of the lungs, which was traced to his refusal to wear a hat or overcoat during his inaugural address.

A NEW SUSPECT—BACTERIA

In the middle of the nineteenth century, a French professor of chemistry, Louis Pasteur, discovered a clue that pointed the way toward the true cause of colds and flu. Officials from the French wine industry approached Pasteur for help in finding the cause of some unwanted by-products that were forming during their fermentation process. At that time, it was assumed that the yeast that converted sugar into alcohol was a nonliving chemical.

Pasteur guessed that yeast was a microorganism, and his experiments confirmed this. During these experiments, Pasteur proposed the startling theory (known as the "germ theory") that such microorganisms as bacteria and protozoans played an active role in our world. In fact, he believed that they caused disease in humans. Although the existence of these minute creatures had been demonstrated nearly two hundred years earlier by the invention of the microscope, no one had suspected that these tiny microbes were actually among the most deadly enemies of mankind.

Pasteur's theory was too startling for many medical

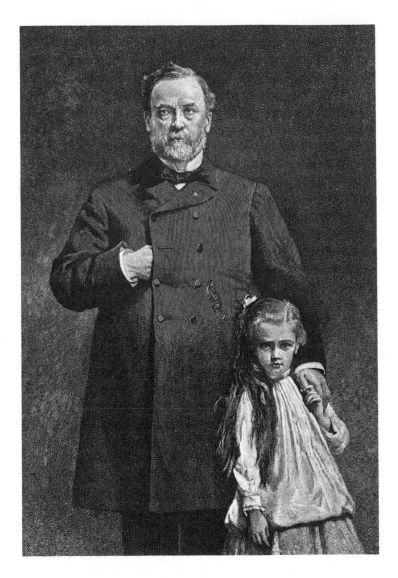

Louis Pasteur (1822–1895), shown here with his granddaughter. The great French scientist postulated the "germ theory," which states that microorganisms can be potent agents of disease.

experts to believe. But the evidence that Pasteur produced sparked the curiosity of German country physician Robert Koch. An ingenious young man who was basically self-trained in microbiology, Koch produced many advances in that field. None was more important than his demonstration that rod-shaped bacteria caused the disease anthrax in animals. Koch's announcement of this in 1876 sent other scientists scurrying to their microscopes. By following Koch's meticulous ground rules for linking microorganisms with a specific illness, researchers discovered, during the 1880s and 1890s, the hidden cause of one disease after another. Tiny bacteria and one-celled organisms called protozoans appeared to be responsible for a great deal of suffering in the world.

German researcher Richard Pfeiffer believed that the flu was one such malady caused by bacteria. In the 1890s, he discovered great numbers of one particular bacteria in the throat of every flu patient he examined. There seemed to be little doubt that the bacterium, named Pfeiffer's bacillus, was the likely cause of flu.

A TINY, LIVING POISON

At about the time of Pfeiffer's work, however, other scientists were finding that the microscopic world was a great deal more crowded than anyone had imagined. Russian researcher Dmitri Ivanoski was the first to stumble across evidence that bacteria might not be the smallest living things on our planet.

It happened while he was investigating a disease that attacked tobacco plants. Following the examples of other scientists of his time, Ivanoski searched for a bacterium or protozoan that might be responsible. He devised an experiment to test the infecting ability of bacteria. He crushed infected tobacco leaves to extract the sap, and then ran the liquid through a filter. The pores of this filter

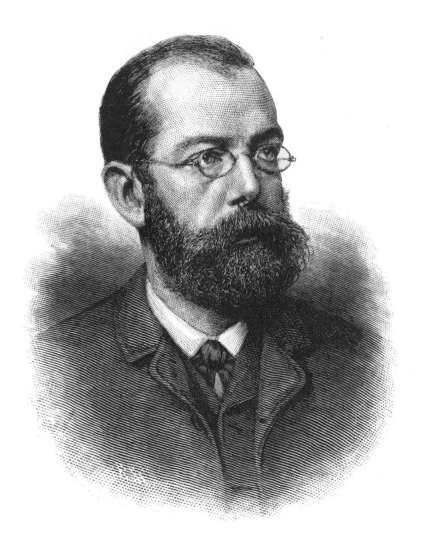

German physician and bacteriologist
Robert Koch (1843–1910) identified a bacteria
as the cause of anthrax, an animal disease.
Koch also studied the tubercle bacillus,
which causes tuberculosis. He was awarded
the Nobel Prize for Medicine in 1905.

were so small that even the smallest bacterium would be unable to pass through.

Ivanoski then injected tobacco leaves with either filtered or unfiltered solutions. If, as expected, the unfiltered sap caused the leaves to be infected and the filtered sap did not, that would be a strong indication that bacteria were responsible for the disease. Instead, as Ivanoski reported in a 1892 paper, the filtered sap retained the ability to infect tobacco leaves as readily as did the unfiltered sap. The apparent conclusion, that some mysterious substance far smaller than bacteria was causing the disease, was too unsettling even for the man who performed the experiments. Ivanoski second-guessed his own experiment and wondered if bacteria had somehow passed through the filter. Given Ivanoski's doubts, it is not surprising that his experiment was largely ignored. Before long, however, other researchers came up with the same odd results when they tried to filter bacteria from disease-causing solutions. In 1898, the German researchers Loffler and Frosch discovered that hoof-and-mouth disease in cattle could be produced by supposedly bacteria-free solutions taken from infected beasts.

A year later Dutch botanist Martinus Beijerinck, who was unfamiliar with Ivanoski's work, performed an experiment similar to that attempted by the Russian. Like Ivanoski, Beijerinck found that liquid steeped from a leaf infected with tobacco mosaic disease could cause the disease in other tobacco leaves even after it was strained free of bacteria. He further observed that if this filtered solution were heated, it lost its power to infect.

The fact that the heat seemed to kill the infecting agent convinced Beijerinck that he had come across some kind of "contagious living fluid." Beijerinck referred to the infecting agent in the liquid as a *virus,* since at that time the term *virus,* from the Latin word for poison, was used as the name for any unknown substance that caused disease.

Within a few years, a growing roster of human diseases, including the deadly yellow fever, had been linked to what were now called "filterable viruses." Since Richard Pfeiffer had previously isolated a bacteria as the cause of influenza, the subject of viruses did not come up in the discussion of upper respiratory diseases for many years. But during the height of the horrible Spanish flu outbreak in 1918, a French physician named Debre began to doubt Pfeiffer's conclusion. Debre noticed that his flu patients reacted to the illness in much the same way as those infected with the measles.

By that time, it had been shown that measles was caused by one of those unseen, filterable viruses. Debre used the same test that Ivanoski had developed to see if Pfeiffer's bacillus was truly responsible for the flu. He ran some blood and pus from an infected patient through tiny, bacteria-trapping filters, and injected the filtered liquid into a subject. The subject developed the flu. Therefore, Debre reasoned, the flu must be caused by a virus.

Debre's analysis was not readily accepted. Filters in use at the time were not always reliable, and other scientists attempting the same experiment found that the filtered fluid did not infect the new subject. In the 1920s, a physician at the London Medical School declared that there was "not the slightest shred of evidence that the disease is due to a so-called filter-passing virus."

ZEROING IN ON THE VIRUS

Scientists were groping in the dark throughout the first third of the twentieth century because filterable viruses were almost impossible to study. These infecting agents were too small to be seen even with a microscope. Whereas bacteria could be grown easily in a laboratory, no one had figured out how to grow viruses. No one could say for certain if they could be grown, or if they were even alive. Scientists never were able to isolate or identify the virus responsible for the terrible Spanish flu pandemic.

Slowly, however, the evidence mounted that a filterable virus was the cause of flu. A veterinarian, J.S. Koen, of Fort Dodge, Iowa, noticed a remarkable similarity between the Spanish flu and a disease that was common in pigs. Further research showed this swine flu to be caused by a virus.

All doubt was finally eliminated during the 1930s, when researchers developed the tools that would help them study viruses. In 1931, American scientist W. J. Elford designed a series of filters with tiny pores that were far more carefully calibrated than those ordinarily used. This precise filtering system demonstrated that viruses came in a variety of sizes. Larger viruses could not pass through the bigger pores and so were separated from smaller viruses. Smaller pores then separated small viruses from tiny ones. A number of the viruses known to cause disease could be isolated according to their size.

Other scientists used *centrifuges* rather than filters to separate viruses. The force of a spinning centrifuge would throw heavier viruses to the bottom of the tube. It was one of these centrifuges that first isolated the virus responsible for influenza.

An American researcher named Wendell Stanley was the first to find out what these filterable viruses were. He became convinced that viruses were made of protein, and he designed an ambitious experiment to test his theory. In order to get all the material he needed for his experiment, Stanley extracted the juice from a ton of tobacco leaves infected with mosaic disease. He then chemically separated all the protein from the solution. Stanley then rubbed some of this protein paste on healthy tobacco leaves. Sure enough, they developed tobacco mosaic. From this, Stanley concluded that viruses were made up of protein. A few years later, he discovered that he had not been entirely right. Viruses were found to contain a small amount of *nucleic acid* as well as protein.

Nucleic acid and protein are common molecules in living things. Yet when Stanley examined his extracted protein, he found that it formed long, jagged crystals. No living organism was known to take on the shape of a crystal. Stanley concluded that viruses were a different form of organism, neither completely live nor dead. He referred to them as being "in the twilight zone of life."

At about the time when Stanley was discovering the chemical nature of viruses, other scientists were solving the frustrating problem of how to grow and study living, active viruses.

In the mid-1930s, London laboratory workers observed that ferrets, unlike other animals, seemed to develop flu symptoms during an outbreak of flu among humans. This was confirmed when ferrets injected with fluids from an infected human developed flu symptoms. By itself, this knowledge was of little practical value to scientists. While a few tests could be run using ferrets, no laboratory could afford the expense of keeping a huge supply of such animals for research.

Some of the ferrets, however, developed serious lung infections from their *inoculation*. This was bad for the ferrets but good for virus research. The discovery that a virus could grow on lung tissue led to the culturing of viruses in the lungs of smaller, more affordable animals, such as mice. Eventually, an even better method of growing viruses was discovered. Viruses were found to grow well when injected into eggs containing live chick embryos. Viruses used to develop vaccines today are commonly grown inside live eggs. *Virologists,* those who specialize in the study of viruses, have also perfected techniques of growing viruses on cells in test tubes and bottles.

Another tool that greatly aided virus research was the electron microscope, developed around 1930. Ordinary

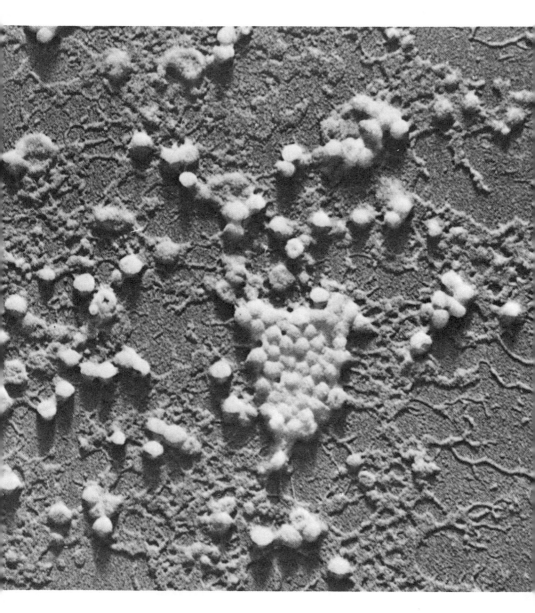

A magnified view of influenza virus
type B taken with an electron microscope.
The individual viruses appear to be round.

microscopes focus light on the object to be viewed. If the object is much smaller than the wavelength of the light used, the object cannot be made visible. Viruses are in this category and so cannot be viewed under a conventional microscope. The electron microscope, however, focuses a beam of electrons, minute subatomic particles, on the object. Electron microscopes, able to magnify an object 100,000 times, finally presented a glimpse of the filterable "poison" that Beijerinck had spoken of half a century earlier.

With these new tools of research, scientists confirmed that the virus was indeed responsible for a great deal of human suffering, including smallpox, polio, and influenza. In the early 1940s, researchers added the common cold to that list. By that time, however, colds and flu had been so firmly linked with exposure to drafts and cold weather that the notion was difficult to dislodge from popular belief.

3

VIRAL WARS

Many people still speak of viruses as though they were mysterious, invisible menaces with unknown, almost magical powers. When no other explanation can be found for an illness, the problem is usually blamed on "some kind of virus." Nothing more is said about it, as if viruses were outside the realm of knowledge.

In fact, scientists know a great deal about viruses and how they make us miserable. A virus is the simplest living thing that inhabits our world, so simple that the debate has never been resolved as to whether it is really alive at all. Some of the hardier viruses can exist for years without functioning in any way, looking and acting for all the world like a nonliving molecule.

The largest virus is about one-third the size of the smallest bacteria. The smallest ones are so tiny that more than 200 million of them would fit inside the period at the end of this sentence. Cold and flu viruses are on the smaller end of the scale.

A virus is composed of a tiny packet of genetic material enclosed in a shell made up of four proteins. This genetic material, known as nucleic acid, comes in the form of either DNA or RNA, which are the master molecules that control the functions of all living cells. Viruses, how-

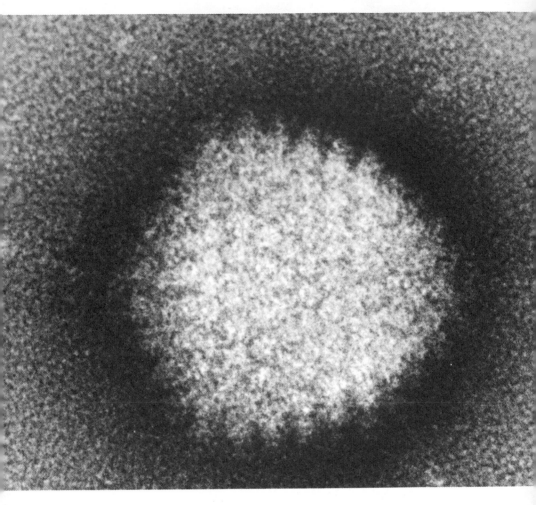

Above: Magnified view of adenovirus, one of the six different families of cold-causing viruses. The virus contains double-stranded DNA surrounded by a protein capsid (coat). The capsid is composed of "capsomers," which appear as tiny ovals.
Facing page: Adenoviruses as seen under lower magnification

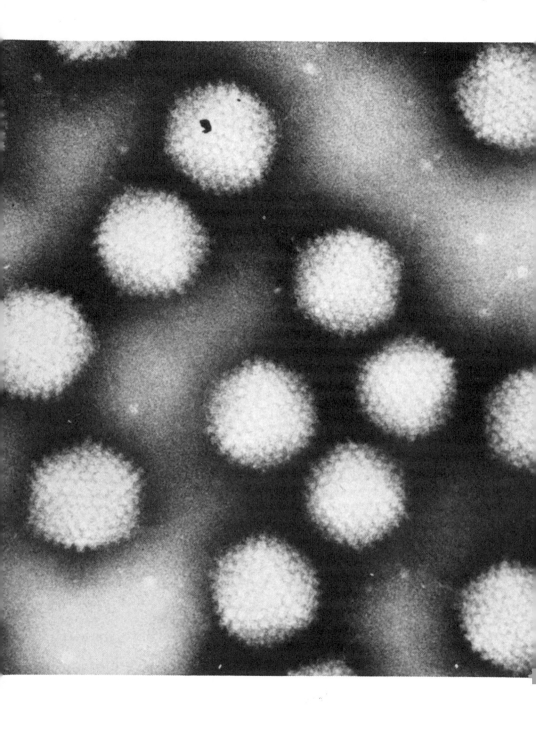

ever, contain no functional parts for the nucleic acid to direct. Unlike all other living things, viruses are not capable of reproducing themselves. They are parasites who must borrow reproductive equipment from other living organisms in order to multiply.

Viruses have been remarkably successful in carrying out their parasitic existence, and they are known to attack virtually every species of living thing. Not all of these submicroscopic entities are harmful. But none of them has been found to have any useful purpose that humans can appreciate, and many of them have proven particularly dangerous to their hosts. Several families of viruses find exactly what they need for rapid reproduction in the cells that line the human nose and throat. These viruses are the causes of colds and flu.

Only three types of viruses, from a single family, are responsible for influenza. Viral rhinitis, the common cold, is a far more complicated matter, so complicated that the illness posed a mystery to researchers long after the causes of most other common diseases had been found. When the mystery was finally unraveled, it was no wonder that researchers had been so baffled. Scientists have come to discover that roughly 200 different viruses, from six different families, produce illnesses that are so similar to one another that they are all lumped together in the category of colds. About half of these cold-causing viruses are of a similar type and are known as *rhinoviruses* (rhino means nose). Other cold-causing viruses include the coronaviruses and adenoviruses. None of the cold-causing viruses is known to attack any other organism besides humans.

ATTACK OF THE COLD VIRUS

Cold viruses reproduce best at between 85 and 95 degrees Fahrenheit. Since human body temperature is slightly higher than that, the cold virus is most likely to

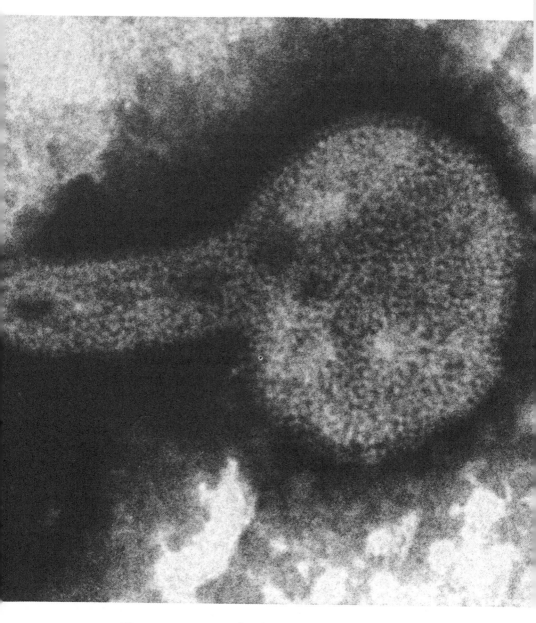

Electron micrograph of Hong Kong flu virus
as seen under very high magnification

infect one of the cooler portions of the respiratory system—one of the passages that leads outside the body. Viruses that cause infection usually enter through the nose or the tear ducts. Experiments have shown that live cold viruses introduced into the mouth rarely cause a cold, while similar viruses placed in the nose or the eyes consistently result in illness.

Viruses cannot move by themselves, and so they have to be carried to these points of infection. There are two ways that viruses can be transported to a nasal passage: they can be propelled through the air by a sneeze, a cough, or exhaling, or they can be transferred from one place to another by direct contact.

Researchers have not resolved the debate over which of these two methods is most responsible for spreading colds. In 1973, Owen Hendley and Jack Gwaltny of the University of Virginia showed that the hands of cold victims are teeming with viruses, and that some of these viruses are transferred to nearly everything the person touches. Hendley and Gwaltny gave fifteen healthy student volunteers the disgusting task of rubbing on their hands nasal discharge from those with colds. Eleven of the fifteen developed colds. Meanwhile, only two of twelve students who just sat at a table with cold sufferers got sick.

From this, Hendley and Gwaltny concluded that the majority of colds are passed along through touch. A person suffering from a cold touches an infected area by wiping his or her nose or eyes, and then transfers the virus to the next thing he or she touches. Cold viruses can survive on cloth, telephone surfaces, doorknobs, cups, plates, and silverware for hours, ready to infect the next person who makes contact with those items.

Other scientists cite experiments by Elliot Dick of the University of Wisconsin in which it was demonstrated that cold viruses were not transferred by direct contact. Dick had a group of healthy students play poker with cards

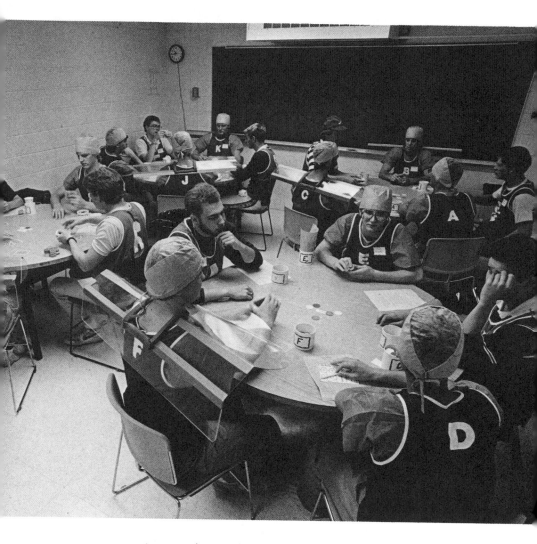

In a study conducted at the University of Wisconsin at Madison, one group of students played poker using cold-virus-contaminated cards and chips while another group played poker with cold victims. The results indicated that airborne viruses are the primary means of transmission.

that were soggy from contamination with nasal secretions of cold sufferers. The poker chips and the tables were also contaminated. These students were encouraged to touch their eyes and nose frequently, yet they did not catch colds. Another group of students played poker with cold victims. These students were kept from touching their nose and eyes, yet many of them still got colds. This appears to indicate that a person catches a cold by inhaling viruses that have been expelled into the air by another infected person.

Regardless of which mode of transmission is most responsible, every virus that finds its way into the body presents a potential threat to its new host. Over the course of time, the human body has developed an elaborate, many-layered system of defenses to repel these attacks. The first line of defense consists of *cilia* and mucus. Tiny, hairlike cilia line the nose and throat, capturing dust, dirt, toxins, and germs that are breathed in along with air. Glands inside the lining of the nose manufacture the sticky mucus that traps more of these invaders. A healthy person manufactures as much as a quart of mucus per day. Thanks to this first line of defense, most cold viruses that reach the nose never make it to their intended target. They are either destroyed by the adenoids (folds of tissue behind the nose and mouth) or are washed into the digestive tract where they are killed by stomach acids.

Occasionally, though, a virus gets past this front line of protection and breaks into a cell. Like a pirate boarding a merchant ship, the nucleic acid in the virus immediately takes command of the cell nucleus. Instead of performing its usual functions, the cell nucleus follows the orders given by the viral nucleic acid. Those orders are simple: make as many viruses as possible, as quickly as possible. Within hours, the cell is cranking out hundreds of copies of the original virus. Eventually the cell bursts, leaving behind a weakened, damaged, or dead cell and sending thousands of viruses out to infect other cells.

A cold victim does not immediately feel the effects of the viral attack. The time between the initial infection and the first symptoms of a cold is called the "incubation" period. For a cold, the incubation time is generally two or three days. At the latter end of the incubation period, the aggravating effects of the cold take hold gradually. Most people can "feel a cold coming on."

THE COUNTERATTACK

Even such a mild illness as a cold would be deadly to humans if the cold virus continued to breed and to destroy cells at its initial pace. But the body is further protected by a vast, intricate immune system. One out of every 100 body cells, roughly one trillion altogether, functions as part of the immune system. These cells can communicate closely with each other to coordinate their counterattack against all invading bacteria, protozoans, viruses, or toxins, which are collectively known as *antigens*.

The body's immune system was first observed in action shortly after Pasteur and Koch discovered the role played by bacteria in human diseases. European scientists peering through their microscopes to watch harmful bacteria at work in the human body observed a furious counterattack. Tiny substances in the blood grabbed onto the germs like leeches, and large cells seemed to surround and devour the invading bacteria. The tiny substances were named *antibodies* and the devouring cells were called white blood cells or *phagocytes* (literally "cell-eaters").

We now know that these two immune system components patrol all areas of the body. The phagocytes absorb and destroy anything that appears foreign to them, including dead matter as well as antigens. The antibodies are each designed to attack a specific type of antigen. The immune system also includes specialized immune cells, known as *T cells* because they mature in the thymus, a

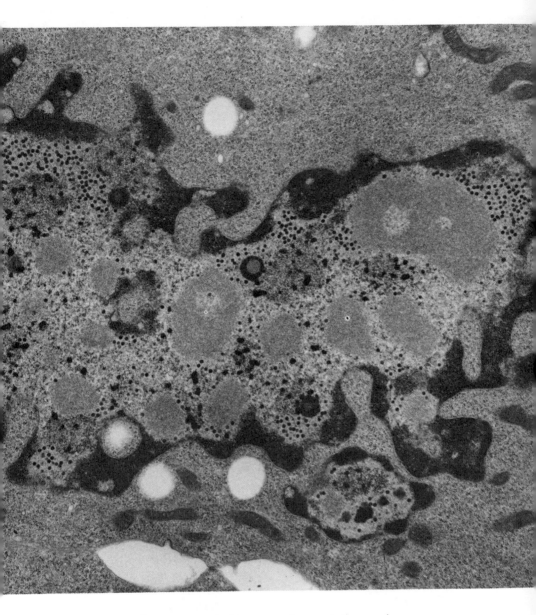

Adenoviruses (white areas) attack the nucleus
of a cell in this image created by a
transmission-electron microscope (TEM).

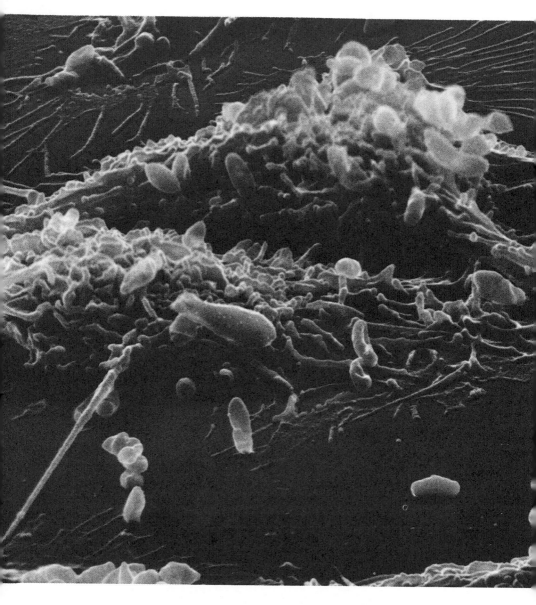

A macrophage engulfs and devours
pseudomonas, a rod-shaped bacteria.
Macrophages are a type of white blood cell.

gland located behind the breastbone. T cells act as scouts. Like the antibodies, they are programmed to recognize a particular antigen.

The body's immune system begins preparing its massive counterattack almost immediately after infection. Phagocytes envelop and kill the viruses they find in the bloodstream. Antibodies latch onto viruses to prevent them from attacking cells, and then hold them until a phagocyte can come to finish off the invader.

A virus particle that has already penetrated a cell, however, is safe from the phagocytes. During the incubation time of a cold or flu, the viruses reproduce far too quickly for the body's normal phagocytes to handle, and the immune system sends out a call for reinforcements. When a T cell happens across a foreign substance that it recognizes, it summons specialized killer T cells to the scene to destroy the invaders. It also signals these killer cells to multiply quickly in order to combat the runaway reproduction of the bacteria.

Unlike white blood cells, killer T cells are able to get at viruses that have already penetrated body cells. They are alerted to the presence of a virus in a cell by a molecule known as *MHC* (for major histocompatibility complex). This molecule captures a tiny piece of the invading virus and holds it up for the T cell to recognize. The T cell then punctures the cell walls so that the viruses spill out where they can be destroyed by both killer T cells and phagocytes.

Meanwhile, cells that have been invaded by viruses release chemicals that bring more of the immune system's reserve forces into the fight. These chemicals attract more large, virus-eating white blood cells, and enlarge the tiny capillaries of the bloodstream so that white blood cells can pass through to the infected area. They also stimulate the production of more antibodies.

Within a couple of days, the massive counterattack launched by the body's immune system begins to take ef-

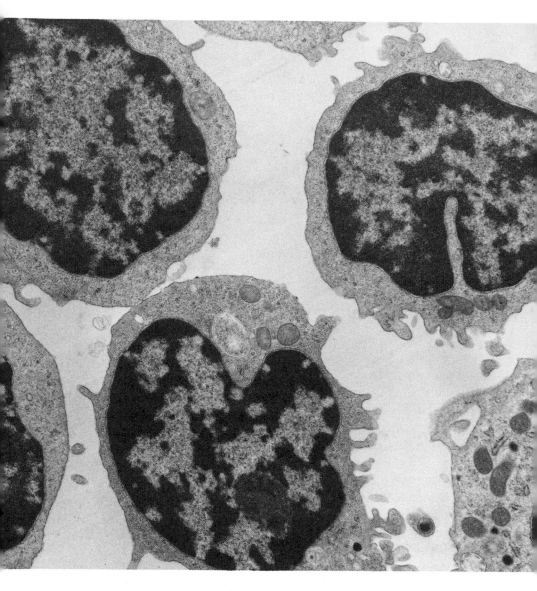

T cells can both
attack viral infections
and regulate other immune
system components.

fect. Most of the familiar cold symptoms that make us miserable are not directly produced by the virus but are the collateral damage of the immune system's effort to defeat the virus. The chemicals released by the damaged cells irritate nerves in the throat, and the result may be a sore throat and perhaps a cough. Some of the chemicals (known as "*histamines*") cause the tissues to swell up, which interferes with the normal draining of fluids. The cold victim experiences this as congestion in the nose, throat, and sinuses. Immune system chemicals also stimulate glands inside the lining of the nose to increase their production of mucus to flush viruses out of the infected areas. This accounts for the most common cold symptoms, a runny nose and dripping in the throat.

On the average, the body's immune system can defeat a cold virus infection in a week. About a quarter of all cold infections may last longer, up to two weeks. Congestion and excess mucus production may linger for a few days beyond the infection, and viruses may be present in the system for several weeks, but by then the battle has essentially been won.

But while the cold viruses almost always lose the battle, they never lose the war. They use the body's own defenses, the runny nose and sneezing, to spread their misery to other battlefronts.

The hit-and-run pattern of colds rarely results in lingering effects for the cold victim. On rare occasions, however, cold viruses spread to other areas of the body, where they cause additional problems. A severe cold virus infection may penetrate to the bronchial tubes, the air passages that branch from the trachea into the lungs. This illness, called *bronchitis*, produces a dry, hacking cough, sore throat, shortness of breath, and fever. Viruses may even penetrate into the lungs to produce viral pneumonia, with symptoms similar to those of bronchitis, only occurring deeper in the chest.

If the virus infects the vocal chords, laryngitis may result, causing a temporary loss of voice. Young children may develop the *"croup"* from a cold virus infection. Symptoms include a short, barking cough and, occasionally, difficulty breathing. Viral infection of the inner ears can cause dizziness and loss of balance.

INFLUENZA ATTACK

A flu virus attacks the upper respiratory tract in much the same way as a cold virus, only the onslaught is usually more intense. Three main types of flu virus have been identified, and they are classified simply as type A, B, and C.

Type A influenza is the most severe, and is responsible for the deadly flu plagues that have swept the world every ten to fifteen years. It is also known to strike birds and various mammals as well as humans. In fact, many researchers believe flu was originally a disease of animals that gradually mutated into a form that could infect humans. The various strains of type A influenza are named according to the location in which they appear to have originated. The devastating *pandemic* of 1918–19 is referred to as the Spanish flu. The 1935–36 pandemic was the London flu, the 1968 outbreak was the Hong Kong flu.

Type B influenza tends to be similar to type A but is far less common. Type C is also rare. Its symptoms are milder than type A and type B and are similar to a cold. Unlike type A flu, B and C can only infect humans.

Flu viruses are spread in the same way as cold viruses, by human interaction either through inhalation of the viruses or possibly by contact. The incubation period for the flu is often shorter than for a cold—only a day or two. As a result, flu can spread very quickly. With airline service carrying people to all parts of the world in just hours, a flu pandemic can sweep many countries in a matter of weeks. The Hong Kong flu, for example, spread rapidly to the United States because it was carried back by American servicemen returning from duty in the Vietnam war.

Flu viruses attack the cells so suddenly that victims rarely feel flu coming on. All at once, the victim develops chills, high fever, aching joints and muscles, severe headache, fatigue, loss of appetite, a cough, and a general feeling of weakness and nausea. Cold symptoms, such as runny nose, sore throat, and congestion are present in about half of flu cases. People often refer to a sudden attack of vomiting and diarrhea as "intestinal flu," but such viral diseases are unrelated to flu.

As with a cold, many of the symptoms of flu are caused by the body's attempt to repel the invaders. The cold symptoms are caused by the same release of chemicals from damaged cells as described earlier. The more intense onslaught of flu viruses prompts the body to take even stronger measures of defense than with a cold. Cells release a protein that signals the brain to raise the body temperature. This increased temperature slows down the rate of viral reproduction and increases the activity of the immune system. In so doing, however, it greatly increases the patient's discomfort.

Other symptoms more common to a flu than a cold, such as headache, aching muscles, chills, and fatigue are believed to result from poisonous products released by the viruses themselves into the bloodstream.

Some cases of influenza may last for several weeks and leave the victim listless for many more days.

SECONDARY EFFECTS

By themselves, colds and flu are miserable nuisances but are not a danger to long-term health. A severe problem, however, may arise because of a secondary bacterial infection.

Congestion and swelling caused by colds and flu can prevent normal drainage of mucus and fluids, and this allows bacteria to grow in the clogged areas. In children this is most likely to occur in the ears and cause earaches. Adults may experience more problems with the sinus cavities that spread out from the nose. The infection known as sinusitis can cause severe headaches and congestion.

Cold and flu viruses may also destroy or damage so many cells and so weaken the natural defenses that the infected areas of the body are left vulnerable to bacterial infections that a healthy person could easily ward off. The most dangerous *secondary infection,* one that is associated with flu far more than colds, is *pneumonia.*

Pneumonia is a general term for any infection and inflammation of the lungs. Three million Americans contract pneumonia each year, and about one-third of sufferers require hospitalization. Once a person has had pneumonia, he or she is susceptible to catching it again. Until the discovery of the bacteria-killing drug penicillin, pneumonia was one of the leading causes of death in the world. Even with effective antibiotics, more than 55,000 deaths occurred from pneumonia in the United States in 1990, making it the sixth leading cause of death. Pneumonia is most dangerous for the elderly, infants, and those with severe heart and lung problems, but it is dangerous to anyone. The sudden death of entertainer Jim Henson, the creator of the Muppets, in 1990, is a grim reminder that pneumonia is still a deadly disease.

4

VACCINATION: DECEPTION AND COUNTER-DECEPTION

Harmful viruses and other microorganisms that infect the body tend to be very successful in their initial attack. As elaborate as the human body's immune system may be, there is simply no way that it can be fully prepared for the arrival of the millions of infective agents that can enter the body. Each of the antibody and T cell "scouts" is programmed to recognize one particular invader. In order to protect against every potential enemy in every area of the body, these scouting forces must be thinly spread out. Antigens that infect a specific area, then, meet only token resistance at first and quickly gain the upper hand.

Only after the attack is in progress does the body's immune system know exactly what it is fighting, and only then can it begin to mount the massive counterattack. Once it has suffered some damage from an invader, however, the immune system is not about to be surprised a second time. It recognizes this particular infecting agent, a virus for example, as a serious threat and takes special precautions to guard against another attack by that organism. The immune system continues to manufacture the specific antibodies that can combat that particular virus.

The next time that type of flu virus enters the body, the immune system is ready for it. Instead of breaking through the token resistance of the scattered phagocytes of antibodies, the invader is crushed by overwhelming force before it gets anywhere. When this happens, the person is said to be immune to the illness.

Physicians have learned to use this fact to artificially arm the immune system against some insidious diseases before they actually strike. In effect, the vaccine injected by the doctor fools the immune system into believing it is under attack so that it will manufacture disease-preventing antibodies that will be used later in the event of a real attack.

The first person to prevent a virus-caused disease through artificial immunization actually knew very little about the immune system. In the late eighteenth century, a British country doctor named Edward Jenner became curious about the disease known as smallpox. Smallpox was one of the most dreaded diseases of the time. Most people contracted smallpox sometime during their lives, and nearly one-third of those infected died. Even those who survived were often left with ugly scars from the pocks that blistered their skin.

Jenner had no idea that smallpox was caused by a virus. The discovery of viruses was still far off in the future, as was the notion that microorganisms could cause disease. Jenner, however, was aware of a common claim among the country folk that milkmaids who contracted a mild disease called cowpox were safe from the far more dangerous smallpox.

Rather than dismissing the idea as superstition, Jenner made his own observations and found that it appeared to be true: milkmaids did not get smallpox. The cowpox that they did contract seemed to Jenner to be very much like a mild case of smallpox, complete with a few small sores on the hands that quickly went away.

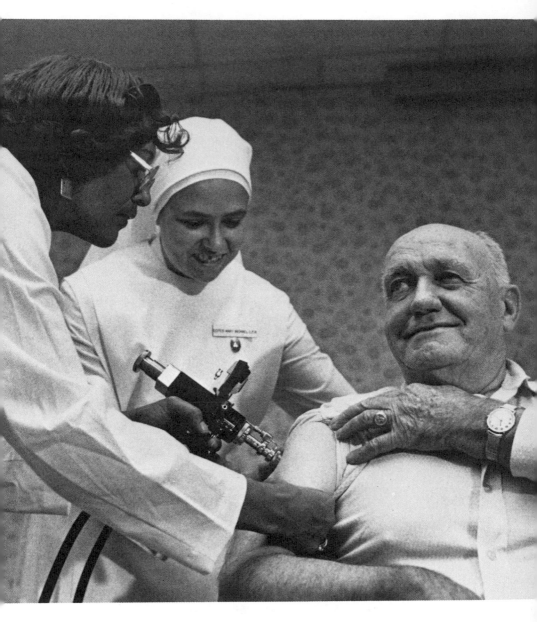

An elderly man receives a flu shot.
The elderly who contract the flu
are vulnerable to serious complications.

It was well established that those who survived a bout with smallpox did not get the disease again. Jenner figured that cowpox must be so closely related to smallpox that a person who was immune to one would also be immune to another.

Jenner became so certain of this that he took a terrible chance, one that would be outlawed by authorities today. Working in a small town in Gloucester, England, Dr. Jenner demonstrated his theory by using an eight-year-old boy as a guinea pig. First, he drew a sample from a sore of a milkmaid infected with cowpox. Then he made two cuts in the arm of young James Phipps and rubbed the infected material into the wound. Not surprisingly, Phipps developed the short-lived sores of cowpox.

Six weeks later Jenner tried to infect Phipps with a deadly illness. He removed some pus from a sore of a smallpox victim and rubbed it into the cuts in the boy's arm. Then they waited to see if Jenner's outrageous gamble worked.

It did. James Phipps did not develop smallpox. He apparently had been made immune to the disease. Jenner referred to what he had done as "*vaccination*," after "*vaccinia*," which is the Latin term for cowpox.

The idea of preventing a serious disease by infecting people with a lesser disease offered a sunburst of hope for a world that had been ravaged by deadly epidemics for centuries. Jenner's technique was widely used to protect people from smallpox, and the once-dreaded disease began to pass into the pages of history. In 1979 the World Health Organization, still using Jenner's basic vaccination method, wiped smallpox from the face of the Earth.

Unfortunately, Jenner's astounding breakthrough turned out to be a fluke. The principle of *cross-reactivity*—of one virus producing an immune reaction against a similar virus—is extremely rare. The antibodies and T cells of the immune system are normally very accurate in their identification of a foreign substance. The 100 million or so different varieties of antibodies and T cells are capable of recognizing every species of bacteria and virus that exist. In fact, these immune components are able to recognize and dispose of laboratory-created chemicals that do not exist in nature!

Jenner happened to stumble upon an exceptional case wherein the immune system mistook a smallpox virus for a cowpox virus. Researchers have found few cases in which they could create immunity by substituting a lesser disease for a greater one. The human immune system appears to be especially specific in attacking cold and flu viruses, and no suitable substitutes have been found.

Jenner's discovery, however, paved the way for further efforts in immunology. Louis Pasteur, working nearly ninety years after Jenner's first immunization, stumbled upon a more promising avenue of disease prevention. Pasteur had been growing a *culture* of chicken cholera bacteria when he interrupted his work to take a vacation. The *cholera* culture was accidentally left out on the shelf.

When Pasteur returned to the laboratory from his vacation two weeks later, he came across the culture. Although he was not certain that the old cholera culture was of any use, he injected a sample of the culture into laboratory animals. As he had feared, none of the animals developed the disease. But then a curious thing happened. He injected the same animals with fresh, potent cholera bacteria, and they still did not contract the disease.

Pasteur explained the situation by proposing that the bacteria that had been left out for two weeks had been so weakened that it was unable to cause the disease, yet it was still strong enough to bring about *immunity*. Following Pasteur's lead, many microbiologists set about to find ways to weaken some of the more deadly infecting agents. They tried heating, freezing, drying, and even breaking up the bacteria.

Pasteur focused much of his work on a disease called rabies. Rabies is transmitted through the bites of animals, and it is almost always fatal to humans. Pasteur believed that some kind of bacteria was responsible for the disease. He discovered that this "bacteria" became far less potent as he transplanted it, as part of infected nerve tissue, from one infected dog to another. He was thus able to cause the bacteria to lose its power to infect.

In 1885, a boy named Joseph Meister was bitten by a rabid dog and brought to Pasteur for treatment. Pasteur's vaccination was designed to prevent rabies, not cure it. But since rabies symptoms do not develop until a couple of weeks after a bite, he hoped there was still time to vaccinate against the disease. With nothing to lose, Pasteur injected the boy with some of his serum, made of weakened rabies virus.

Like his predecessor Jenner, Pasteur had no way of knowing what was actually happening as a result of his vaccination. In fact, rabies was later shown to be caused by a virus, not by the bacteria that Pasteur had supposed. But luck was with the great scientist in this case. Meister never developed the lethal disease.

Pasteur's idea of weakening the infective agent proved to be immensely valuable in the fight against disease, especially after the discovery of viruses. Two of the most serious viral diseases were yellow fever, a mosquito-borne disease that caused devastation in the tropics and occasional epidemics elsewhere, and polio, a disease that crippled young people.

In the 1930s Max Theiler found that yellow fever virus gradually lost its ability to kill laboratory monkeys. After 176 mouse-to-mouse transfers, the virus did not even kill mice. Other researchers built on Theiler's work to develop a vaccine to provide humans protection from this disease.

In the 1940s, a team of American scientists that included Jonas Salk, developed a means of growing the polio virus on tissue other than nerve tissue. Polio viruses grown on this other tissue lost much of their lethal power.

Eventually in the 1950s, polio vaccines were developed using both killed viruses and weakened viruses that could survive in the intestine but could not invade the nervous system. (Killed viruses are preferred because of the dangers of working with any live virus.) Since that time, virologists have found ways to break up viruses and to make vaccines using very small pieces of viruses.

As more knowledge was gained about viruses, it became clear why all these virus vaccines work: They blow the cover off the disease-causing virus before it has a chance to attack. The virus introduced by the vaccine is too weak to cause much damage to the body's cells, yet it triggers the production of antibodies that combat that virus. If, at some later time, the real, deadly form of the virus penetrates the body's outer defense, the immune system will recognize it and immediately thwart the attack with its built-up defenses.

Since both influenza and colds are caused by viruses, scientists hoped to find a way to build up the body's immunity to them in the same way as with polio and yellow fever. But in its long-standing battle against nature's most advanced life-form, nature's most primitive life-form has proven amazingly resourceful. Both flu and cold viruses have developed strategies to thwart the efficiency of the immune system.

The problem with the flu virus is that it is unstable. Instead of its genetic material being passed on to the next generation intact, the *nucleic acids* in the virus may undergo a significant change from one generation to the next. This means that the flu virus that attacks today may be quite different from its ancestor that infected the same person years ago. The body's immune system may have produced antibodies and built up defenses in response to the original illness, but these defenses will not recognize and, therefore, be unable to destroy, the altered version of the flu.

Medical researchers keep close tabs on the status of flu virus in the world in order to be able to counter the virus's ability to mutate. The U.S. Centers for Disease Control monitors flu reports from all over the world to try to anticipate any new outbreaks and to detect major shifts in the flu virus. Along with scientists from the National Institutes of Health and the Federal Drug Administration, they advise drug manufacturers of current strains so that modified versions of flu vaccine can then be rushed into production.

Predicting the behavior of something as unstable as a flu virus is far from an exact science. An outbreak of swine flu among U.S. Army recruits at Fort Dix, New Jersey, in 1976, sparked great alarm among medical experts. The flu virus appeared to be similar to the one that caused nearly half a million deaths in the United States in 1918. Health authorities geared up for a massive vaccination program to head off the potentially deadly pandemic. The United States ended up spending an enormous amount of money to combat a flu virus that turned out to be far less dangerous than first predicted.

Flu vaccines, however, do save lives. Scientists prepare vaccines by growing, in fertilized eggs, the current strains of the most threatening flu viruses. They then remove the virus-infected fluid from the egg and inactivate it with formaldehyde. This killed virus is then given to people in the form of a flu shot.

The body's immune system responds to this false attack by producing antibodies against that virus. In most cases, it takes about two weeks for the body's defenses to build up enough protection to prevent a real attack from a live version of the virus. Because of the fluctuating nature of flu strains, a flu shot is usually effective for about a year.

A flu shot can prevent the onset of flu about 90 percent of the time in a young, healthy person. Even though

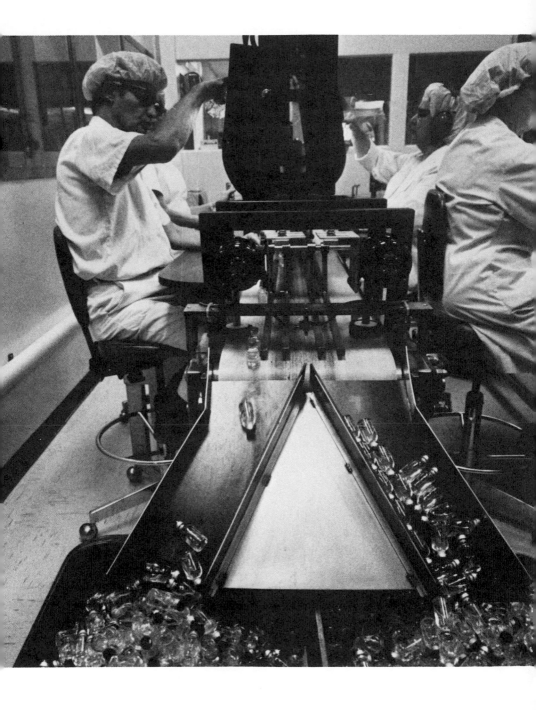

a flu shot works only 70 percent of the time in the elderly, and in those with heart or lung problems, doctors strongly advise them to get flu shots annually, since it is these individuals who are more likely to suffer serious complications as a result of an attack of the flu. Flu shots are also recommended for people who work in health care professions who are in almost constant contact with flu viruses. In spite of doctors' advice, health authorities estimate that only 20 percent of those who could most benefit from flu shots actually receive them.

Currently, there is no vaccine against the common cold, nor is there any practical way of building up immunity to colds in humans. Individually, a cold virus is a fairly easy target for the immune system. The antibodies that the body produces to defeat a cold virus linger in the system and provide immunity from that virus for at least several years. Cold viruses, however, get around the immune system by their sheer numbers. More than two hundred different viruses have so far been identified as causing colds, and researchers do not claim to have found all of the cold culprits. While these viruses, especially the one hundred or so rhinoviruses, are very similar, there is no cross-reactivity among them. There is just enough variation in their protein coats to confuse the immune system so that immunity to one cold virus does not grant immunity to another cold virus. A person can contract a hun-

Facing page: Vials of swine flu vaccines come off the assembly line at a pharmaceutical plant. In 1976, U.S. health officials were seriously concerned that the swine flu virus would cause a major epidemic and recommended a massive vaccination program for at-risk individuals.

dred different colds in a lifetime, obtain immunity to all of them, and still be vulnerable to more colds.

In order to be completely effective, a cold vaccine would have to contain weakened or killed forms of all the cold viruses. Obviously, this would not be practical, even if all the cold-causing viruses could be identified and packaged into one shot. Furthermore, there is evidence that cold viruses can elude the immune system by changing shape from one generation to the next.

5

PREVENTING COLDS AND FLU: FACTS AND FALLACIES

*B*ecause nearly everyone has had some experience with upper respiratory illness, it is not surprising that there are a great many personal opinions to be heard on the subject of colds and flus. Some ideas about colds have persisted for centuries. Modern researchers are attempting to sort through all the facts and fallacies about colds and flu. They are far from solving all the mysteries of these elusive illnesses, and experts continue to disagree on many points. But the following questions and answers attempt to separate fact from fiction concerning some of the most popular beliefs about the prevention of colds and flu.

Can you catch a cold or the flu from standing out in the cold too long or by running around with wet shoes, clothes, or hair?

No. Both colds and flu are caused by viruses, not by dampness, chills, or prolonged exposure to cold weather.

But can exposure to cold weather or chills, or a drastic drop in the surrounding temperature lower your resistance to the viruses that cause colds and flu?

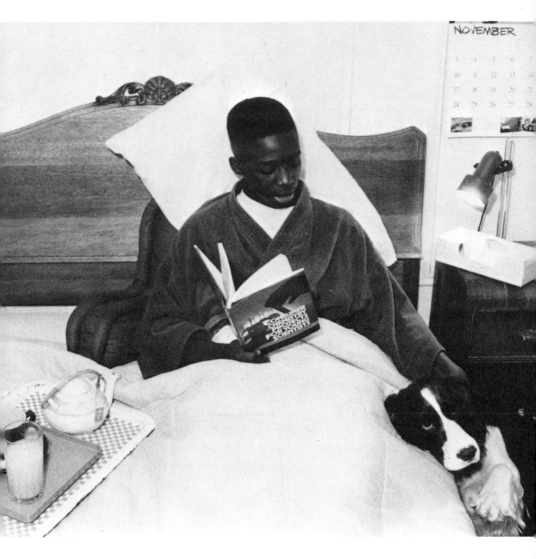

Is bed rest the best prescription for colds and flus? Staying home does prevent the spread of contagion, and certain types of flu can lead to serious complications if you continue your normal routine and give the ailment a chance to linger.

There is not complete agreement among experts. Some physicians believe that subjecting the body to certain kinds of environmental stress may decrease the effectiveness of the immune system. According to a recently published medical guide from England, "a period of exposure to wet and miserable weather may lower your resistance."

Most experts, however, maintain that exposure to drafts and dampness have nothing to do with catching a cold. In an experiment performed at the Common Cold Research Unit in Salisbury, England, in the 1940s, a group of volunteers was soaked with water and then made to stand in a drafty hall for 30 minutes. A second group was kept dry and exposed to a cold virus. A third group was exposed to a cold virus and then given the same wet treatment as the first group. Groups two and three contracted about the same number of colds, while those in group one did not catch colds.

A different research group had poorly clad volunteer test subjects stand in a drafty gymnasium set at 60° F. A second group of volunteers was bundled up and put in a meat locker at 10° F for two hours. A third group was allowed to relax in a comfortably heated room. Live cold viruses were placed in the noses of members of all three groups. Those in the gymnasium who had been thoroughly chilled and those subjected to near freezing weather caught no more nor fewer colds than those who had been in comfortable conditions.

If cold weather is not a factor in causing colds and flu, then why do they occur more often in cold and damp weather?

It is true that people catch colds and flu more often in the winter than in the summer. This is especially true of influenza, which has a definite "season." In the United States, the flu season runs from early December until late March, with a peak period around the beginning of the

New Year. But the reason for this appears to have more to do with people's habits rather than with the weather.

The spread of cold and flu viruses from person to person, either through the air or by direct contact, is far more likely to occur in temperate climates during the colder months. As the weather grows cooler, people spend more time indoors with the windows shut. In late August or September, children go back to school, often to crowded classrooms. Small, enclosed areas with little ventilation are ideal environments for the spread of germs from person to person. The spread of influenza, which is more contagious than the common cold, is highest in the fall and winter months.

During the warmer months in temperate climates, people spend more of their time outdoors and are more likely to keep the windows open in their houses and cars. As a result, there is not as much close, personal contact, and thus there is less chance that disease-causing viruses will be transferred from one person to another.

Dry air may be another cause of the increased number of upper respiratory diseases in the winter months. Dry air can cause the protective mucus to dry up, leaving microscopic, unprotected cracks in the lining of the nasal passage, whose cells viruses find easier to penetrate. Scientists have determined that adding moisture to dry air might prevent colds. A study by Canadian researchers showed that students in schools with high levels of humidity caught 40 percent fewer colds than students in schools with drier air.

Very young children so often seem to have runny noses. Are they more susceptible than older people to colds and flu?

Definitely. Infants and toddlers average more than half a dozen colds per year, and it is not uncommon for a young child to suffer from up to a dozen colds in a year. As people get older, they get fewer colds. Older children may contract four or five colds in a year, teenagers probably average three or four, adults average two or three, and elderly adults average fewer than one per year.

One reason people get fewer colds as they age appears to be natural immunity. The older you get, the better developed your immune system. Also, the more colds you have had, the more cold viruses you are immune to, and so you have less of a chance of catching a cold.

Within the various age groups, are some people more likely than others to catch colds?

Yes. Anyone who spends a great deal of time around children runs a high risk of catching several colds in a year. Children are prime transmitters of cold infections because they catch colds easily, they are less careful about their hygiene, and they spend a great deal of time with each other in classrooms and day care centers, swapping germs.

Women tend to catch more colds than men, primarily because women have more contact with children. Parents of young children catch twice as many colds as adults who do not have children.

People with low incomes have more colds than people with higher incomes. This is thought to occur because people with lower incomes generally live in more crowded conditions.

A small percentage of lucky human beings, estimated at from six to ten percent, never catches a cold at all. This appears to indicate that certain people have exceptionally strong immune systems, and it suggests that one day it may be possible to strengthen the immune system so that it will be able to resist cold viruses.

Is a cold sufferer contagious throughout the course of a cold or only during the initial infection?

A cold or flu victim can be contagious from the moment the viral infection occurs until the last infectious virus is eliminated from the body. But a person is *not* likely to spread a cold during the first stages of infection nor after the symptoms begin to fade. A cold sufferer is most contagious when the symptoms are at their worst, when the nose is constantly runny and sneezing is frequent. These symptoms, which usually reach their peak a few days after the sufferer becomes aware of the cold, spread the virus to a potential point of infection.

Does kissing spread cold and flu germs? What about a glass or cup that the infected person touches with his or her mouth?

The mouth is seldom a source of cold infections. Viruses that attack the upper respiratory system almost always enter the body through the nose and eyes. In a University of Wisconsin study, only one of sixteen volunteers who kissed cold-infected subjects caught a cold.

The mouth has been found to be surprisingly virus-free even during the worst symptoms of an upper respiratory infection, and it is not significantly involved in transmitting cold and flu germs. Cold viruses that enter the mouth are simply swallowed and are destroyed in the stomach. Experiments in which live cold viruses were placed in the mouths of volunteers seldom resulted in a cold. It has been estimated that it takes 1,000 times more rhinoviruses to cause infection through the mouth as through the nose. It is still a good idea, however, not to share a cup or glass with an infected person. There is always the chance you will pick up germs from surfaces the cold sufferer has touched.

Is it better to use a handkerchief or a tissue for blowing your nose?

While a handkerchief may be more stylish than tissues, cold viruses have been shown to survive in a handkerchief for several hours. A tissue used once and thrown away disposes of the contagious viruses immediately and reduces the chance that someone will be accidentally contaminated.

Is there any connection between smoking and upper respiratory diseases?

Yes. Experimental evidence shows that smoking weakens the respiratory system and makes it more vulnerable to infection. People who smoke are especially susceptible to flu-induced pneumonia. Furthermore, studies have shown that children of heavy smokers get colds more frequently than children of nonsmokers.

Does proper diet play any role in preventing respiratory diseases?

Some. Although there are no magic foods that grant immunity from colds and flu, the immune system functions more efficiently when the body is healthy, and an important element of good health is proper nutrition. A person who eats a balanced, sensible diet has a better chance of avoiding colds and of having less severe colds than someone who eats meals with little nutritive value.

Can vitamin C prevent colds?

Maybe. Ever since the first report of the effectiveness of vitamin C in combating colds was published in 1942, the issue has been a source of debate in the medical community. That debate heated up when, in 1970, Nobel Prize-winning chemist Linus Pauling began advocating the use of vitamin C. Vitamin C, also called ascorbic acid, is one of the trace elements and is essential for good health. The vitamin, which is abundant in citrus fruits and many vegetables, has been found to prevent scurvy.

Pauling and many others believe its benefits extend to upper respiratory diseases as well. According to Pauling, "this vitamin exerts a general antiviral action and provides some protection not only against the common cold but also many other diseases, including influenza."

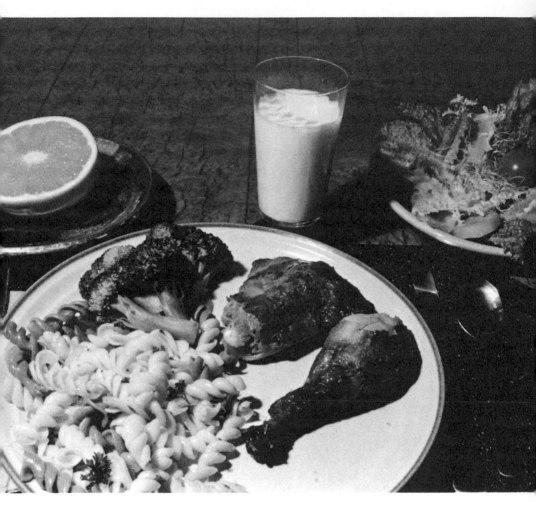

Proper nutrition is a key factor in
maintaining overall health and well-being.

Most in the medical community, however, claim that the vitamin is useless in preventing colds and flu. According to doctors at Columbia University, "Despite popular opinion, it is doubtful that exposed family members or co-workers can gain any protection by taking large amounts of vitamin C."

What are the most effective measures a person can take to avoid catching a cold or the flu?

The best way not to catch a cold or the flu is to stay away from the viruses that cause these illnesses. The only sure way to do that is to avoid infected people as much as possible. Since you don't always know who has a cold or the flu and who does not, it is virtually impossible to avoid the viruses all the time, unless you are a hermit. But you can reduce your chances of catching a cold by shunning crowds, especially when colds and flu are prevalent. Such peopled places as elevators, automobiles, meeting rooms, nurseries, day care centers, offices, and doctors' waiting rooms are prime places for the spread of viruses.

Even if you could isolate yourself from all strangers, however, there is a good chance you will catch a cold anyway. Colds and flu are commonly transmitted from one family member to another in the home. Studies have shown that when one person in a family gets a cold, the other family members have a 40 percent chance of getting that cold.

There are some drastic steps you could take to avoid being infected at home by a family member. For instance, you could wear a mask or have a special air filter installed. But except for elderly people in poor health, and those with heart or respiratory diseases, going to such lengths to avoid catching a mild cold would not be worth the trouble or expense.

Probably the most sensible measure to take when family members have colds is to avoid their sneezes and breathing by giving them a wide berth. Since viruses can survive for many hours on hard surfaces, care should be taken to avoid touching things that have been handled by a cold or flu victim. An infected family member should have his or her own washcloth, towel, cup, and toothpaste tube. Shared objects, such as doorknobs, faucet handles, and telephones should be washed frequently with disinfectant. One study indicated that the chances of catching a cold in the home could be cut by 40 percent with liberal use of a strong disinfectant. Those not infected should wash their hands frequently with soap and water. Even just a quick spurt of water will usually wash off the viruses.

Living in a moist, smoke-free environment can help reduce the chances of catching a cold or the flu. A humidifier can provide the moisture that many houses lack during the cold winter months. But it must, however, be cleaned often, otherwise it could become a prime breeding ground for the very germs you are trying to avoid. Green plants give off moisture and are a safer way of bringing humidity into the home.

You can lessen the chance of catching a cold or the flu by taking care of your health. This includes getting enough rest, eating well, and exercising to keep your body fit, thus enabling it to fight off infection.

Finally, influenza can be prevented by a flu shot, which should be administered once a year at least two weeks before the start of the late-autumn flu season.

What steps should I take to avoid passing along my cold or flu to others?

Common sense tells you to avoid touching your nose. But it is just as important to keep your fingers away from your eyes, even if your eyes are watery. Wash your hands frequently just in case you forget. When you use a tissue, do not save it to use a second or third time; throw it away immediately, and wash your hands. Cover your mouth when coughing, your nose when sneezing, and keep a safe distance from people while conversing.

Again, it is best to avoid close contact with other people as much as possible.

Does this mean you should stay home from school every time you have a cold?

Colds are a nuisance, but life does not have to stop for you each time you get one. However, a classroom is an ideal place to transmit colds and flu. In many cases, transmission of illness could be avoided if sick people would stay home rather than pass along their germs to others. Type A flu can lead to dangerous complications, and those suffering from it should definitely stay at home until the illness runs its course.

6

TREATING COLDS AND FLU: FACTS AND FALLACIES

Not all colds and flu are equally severe, and it is tempting for people to make a connection between an unusually mild illness and some new remedy they tried. This connection may help explain the large number of bizarre treatments that have been prescribed for colds and flu over the years. Even so, it is hard to imagine how a Roman writer, nearly two thousand years ago, came up with the remedy "kissing the hairy muzzle of a mouse."

Up until the last few centuries, many recommended treatments for illness have probably been as harmful as the illness itself. One of the many notable examples of worthless remedies was the treatment given to George Washington after he contracted a cold in December of 1799. Washington was made to gargle with a mixture of molasses, vinegar and butter, and had a preparation made from dried beetles placed on his throat. His doctors also believed that the poisons causing his illness could be drained by "bleeding." Washington was bled four times. He died two days after he became sick.

While the practice of bleeding patients with upper respiratory illnesses has long since ended, a great deal of confusion remains concerning the best ways to treat colds and flu. The following questions and answers attempt to separate fact from fiction concerning some of the most popular beliefs about cold and flu remedies.

Is there any truth to the common saying that the best treatment in the world will cure a cold in about a week while a cold left to run its course may linger for as long as seven days?

Yes. The facetious statement emphasizes the point that most cold remedies relieve only the symptoms of a cold and do nothing to cure the illness. There is, in fact, no widely accepted "cure" for the common cold.

On the other hand, there are a number of measures that can be taken to help an immune system fight a viral infection. Doctors recommend that a person with a viral infection get plenty of rest. There is usually no need to stay in bed because of a cold, but failure to take it easy may cause the illness to linger, may weaken the body's efforts to fight off serious secondary bacterial infections, or even cause inflammation of the heart.

Is it difficult to distinguish a cold from an allergy?

It can be. An allergic reaction is caused by an overprotective immune system. When such harmless particles as pollen and dust are inhaled into the upper respiratory tract, the immune system reacts to them as though they are dangerous antigens. The antibodies sound a false alarm, causing the cells to release a chemical that produces the familiar antigen-flushing mechanisms.

Allergy symptoms are often identical to those of a cold and may include congestion; runny nose and dripping in the throat; watery, itchy eyes; and, occasionally, a headache. Allergies may even bring on a few of the same complications as a cold, such as sinusitis.

Circumstances often will make clear the difference between an allergy and a cold. If the same symptoms keep occurring at the same time of year, it is probably due to an allergy caused by some seasonal element of nature, such as tree pollen, hay, and ragweed. Other allergies can be traced to a specific place. For example, if you are allergic to cat dander, you will have the symptoms every time you visit people who have a cat. If you "catch a cold" every time you dust or sand wood, it is almost certainly an allergic reaction. Colds usually clear up within a week or two, so if coldlike symptoms linger for weeks, you may be allergic to something in your own house. If the symptoms are caused by something with which you randomly come in contact, a particular food, for example, distinguishing allergy from cold may be more difficult.

Since the symptoms are so similar, are colds and allergies treated the same way?

Not exactly. In an allergic reaction, the runny nose and dripping in the throat are produced by a protein called histamine. Drugs known as *antihistamines* can keep cells from releasing histamine, and so relieve the allergy symptoms. Since there is no real illness associated with the allergy, the antihistamine can effectively halt the condition.

For many years it was assumed that the runny nose or dripping in the throat and itchy, watery eyes that develop during a cold or the flu were caused by the release of this same protein by the tissues during a viral attack. Working under that assumption, doctors recommended that those who needed relief from a runny nose or dripping in throat use an antihistamine, which is contained in most cold medications that claim to relieve a runny nose.

Recently, however, researchers have uncovered evidence that histamine may not be a factor in the cause of cold or flu symptoms. Two other substances, *interferon* and *bradykinin*, are released by cells under attack by viruses. These chemicals, which trigger an increase in blood flow to the nose, appear to play a far greater role than histamine in causing the typical cold symptoms. If histamine does not cause cold and flu symptoms, then an antihistamine has no effect in alleviating those symptoms.

Furthermore, the excess nasal secretions help the body defend itself against a cold virus. Many doctors think this process should be allowed to take place, and they recommend tolerating a runny nose rather than taking a cold remedy.

Last year, Americans spent more than two billion dollars on over-the-counter cold medications, such as those that include antihistamines. Do any of these products really work, or are they all just a waste of money?

There are no cold medications that can cure a cold or the flu or even help your body fight against these illnesses. The antibiotics that are so effective in wiping out bacteria do not destroy viruses.

Many cold medications have shown some effectiveness, however, in relieving cold symptoms. Although these symptoms are a part of the process that helps the body ward off infection, relief from the misery of cold symptoms is often desirable, particularly when symptoms interfere with sleep or the ability to perform necessary tasks.

Aside from antihistamines, whose effectiveness is questionable, there are three main types of medication to choose from in combating a cold. Each is designed to relieve a specific symptom: congestion, cough, or sore throat.

Decongestants not only relieve stuffiness, but can ease the clogging that could lead to sinusitis. They come in the form of liquid, tablet, and sprays. Nasal sprays are most effective at rapidly relieving congestion. They should not be used for more than a few consecutive days, however, or they can cause more discomfort than the original cold.

Cough and sore throat medications come in liquid or lozenge form. Over-the-counter cold remedies are generally recognized as safe, and so cold sufferers can choose among the various products for what works best for their particular symptom and for the best value.

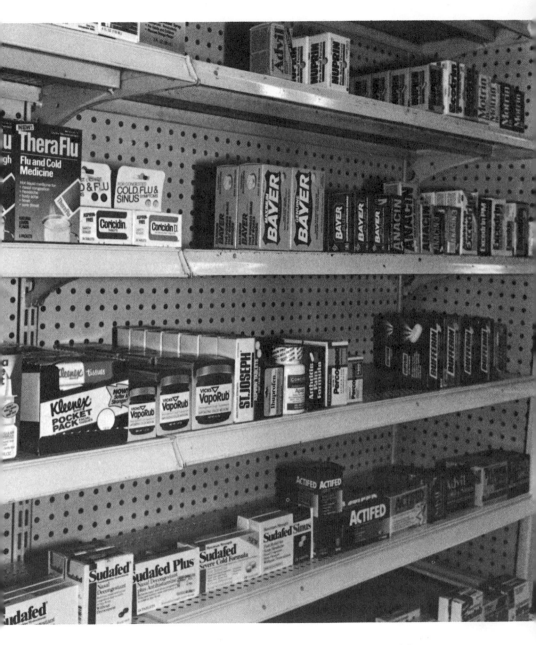

Over-the-counter medications do not cure colds
and flus; they merely alleviate certain symptoms.

Medical experts do not, however, recommend the use of a cold medicine that combines all the symptom-fighting ingredients in one remedy. Although it may seem like less of a hassle to take a single medicine to relieve all of the symptoms, cold symptoms often appear one after another rather than all at the same time. So, with a combination product, you are often paying for medications you do not need. Some remedies cause drowsiness, an unnecessary nuisance if you do not actually need that ingredient. It is cheaper, safer, and more effective to take one specific medication for each cold symptom as it appears.

Does chicken soup do anything for a cold, or is it just another old folk remedy?

Chicken soup is one home remedy that really works. One of the reasons, simply, is that all liquids soothe a sore throat. Liquids also tend to thin out the mucus, which helps the body flush out the infection and relieve congestion that may lead to more serious complications. Furthermore, a hot liquid like chicken soup can raise the body temperature, which inhibits virus *replication* and aids the immune response.

But chicken soup apparently has a special power to relieve congestion beyond that of ordinary liquids, although no one knows exactly how it does this. In one experiment, cold sufferers were fed either cold water, hot water, or chicken soup. Chicken soup was found to clear the nasal passages much better than either of the other liquids tested.

What about those strong-smelling ointments that have been around for decades? Do they work, or are they also just part of folk medicine?

Eucalyptus, camphor, and menthol are some commonly used cold remedy ingredients that pack a powerful aroma. They have been shown to be effective in clearing congested air passages and quieting a cough to allow a more restful sleep.

Lemon and honey is another old-fashioned cold remedy.
Does it help a cold?

Maybe. Lemons are a rich source of vitamin C. As mentioned earlier, the effect of vitamin C on respiratory illness is a controversial subject in the medical community. There does seem to be some evidence that vitamin C can reduce the severity and length of a cold, but whether that evidence is significant or not has been a subject of debate.

Since World War II, there have been more than thirty studies examining the effect of vitamin C on colds. Slightly more than half of them show that the vitamin helps reduce the duration of a cold by as much as 40 percent. A 1989 study conducted at the University of Wisconsin found that cold sufferers taking 2,000 mg of vitamin C per day had colds that were half as severe as those of people taking a *placebo*. (A placebo is a medicine that has no active ingredients.) Many other studies show vitamin C to have no effect on a cold.

Vitamin C supporters point out the flaws in the experiments that show no effect; skeptics say the experiments are faulty that show the vitamin to be beneficial. In experiments in which vitamin C was successful, it was given more frequently and in a stronger dosage. These experiments indicate that a cold will be less severe and of shorter duration if a person begins taking 10 to 20 times the recommended minimum daily requirement of vitamin C at the very first sign of cold symptoms, and continues that dosage until the cold is gone. At this time, there seems to be no harm in taking vitamin C to alleviate cold symptoms. No significant dangers have been associated with ingesting large quantities of the vitamin. Ask your doctor for his or her opinion about vitamin C.

How effective are vaporizers and steam baths?

Moist air serves a number of purposes. It keeps the mucus lining from drying, eases congestion, and keeps the throat from drying out when the nasal passages are too clogged to allow breathing through the nose. Inhaled steam can raise the temperature inside the nose and throat, which inhibits viral reproduction. In severe cases of croup where breathing is difficult, steam inhalation is especially useful in opening air passages.

What effect does alcohol have on a cold or flu?

Alcoholic beverages have been used as a remedy for illness for centuries. A recently published book on family health states that "antibiotics will not help but a tot of whiskey may" in the treatment of colds.

In reality, alcohol provides no benefit for an upper respiratory illness and may do some harm. Alcohol dehydrates the body at a time when it needs all the fluids it can get. It also is known to hamper production of white blood cells and retard the activity of the immune system. Excessive use of alcohol also leaves a flu sufferer more prone to pneumonia.

How accurate is the old saying "feed a cold, starve a fever?"

Not very. Good nutrition is important in combating all kinds of sickness. While a flu victim who runs a high fever may not be up to eating big meals, there is no medical value in denying food to someone who wants to eat.

Should a person with a cold or flu see a doctor?

Usually, there is no need to see a doctor. The body can fight off most colds and flu without medical intervention, and there is nothing a doctor can prescribe that will make any difference.

When a secondary infection develops, however, a doctor should be seen. Symptoms of a secondary infection are an earache, a fever or sore throat that lasts more than a couple of days, or a lingering cough.

The sore throat is the condition that bears the closest

watching, because it can be a symptom of a bacterial infection as well as of a viral infection. Normally, the sore throat that accompanies a cold is not a cause for concern and will go away without treatment. But if the pain persists or is accompanied by more severe symptoms, such as fever, a doctor should be seen. *Strep throat,* an infection caused by the streptococcal bacterium, is often difficult to distinguish from an ordinary, viral-induced sore throat, and cannot be diagnosed for certain without a throat culture. If a strep throat is not treated with antibiotics, heart or kidney damage could result.

What is the most effective treatment for a cold?

It sounds repetitious, but the best way to treat a cold is to get ample rest, drink plenty of fluids, and treat the symptoms with medication only as needed. Rest allows the body to put most of its energy into fighting the infection. Fluids ease congestion, soothe the throat, and prevent dehydration.

What is the best treatment for flu?

Since the flu is usually a more severe illness than a cold, rest and fluids are even more important for flu sufferers than for cold sufferers. The high fever that often accompanies the flu may be treated with damp washcloths or by a sponge bath. A nonaspirin pain reliever can neutralize a headache and help combat a fever. Aspirin can do the same but is not recommended for children with the flu. Aspirin has been linked to a secondary condition, known as *Reye's syndrome,* which sometimes follows type B flu and is dangerous to children.

7

THE FUTURE OF COLDS AND FLU

*F*or years scientists have been cautioning us against getting our hopes up that the common cold would ever be banished from our lives as were other viral diseases, such as smallpox and polio. The constantly changing 200 or so viruses responsible for colds have overwhelmed all known methods of immunization. The fact that viruses cannot be destroyed by penicillin and other bacteria-killing drugs has thwarted all attempts at effective treatment.

Nevertheless, scientists continue to probe the mysteries of cold and flu viruses. Recently, they have uncovered a number of exciting leads that may yet give humans the upper hand in this continuing battle between the most advanced creation of nature and the most primitive. Scientists are taking several paths in their quest for a more cold-free world, and they all involve the body's immune system.

RECEPTOR BLOCKING

Widespread concern over the viral disease known as AIDS has sparked a flurry of research into the ways viruses work and how the body's immune system responds

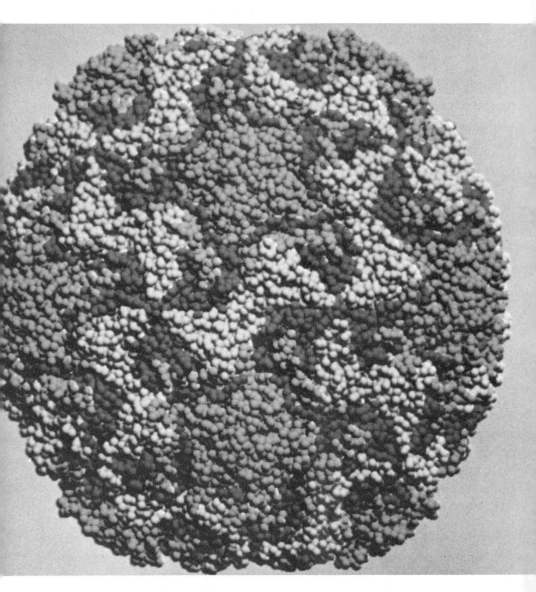

A computer-simulated model of human
rhinovirus-14, which causes colds,
created by a Purdue University research
team led by Dr. Michael Rossman

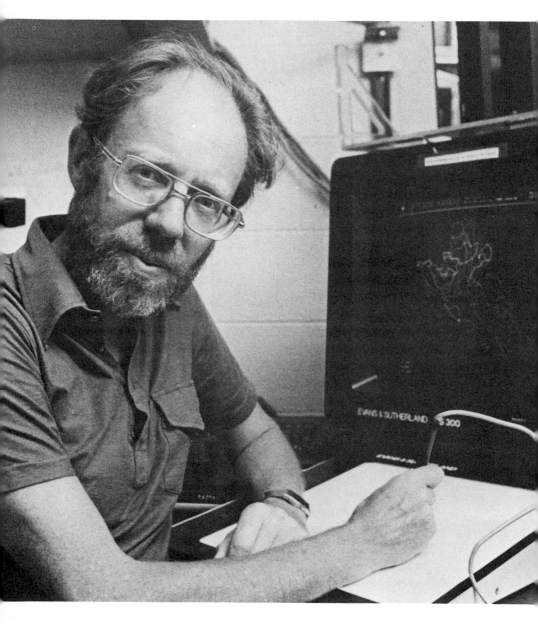

Dr. Rossman with another
one of his simulations

to attack. In 1981, molecular biologist Michael Rossman of Purdue University set out to reproduce an exact model of a cold virus. It was a mind-boggling project. A tiny cold virus contains more than 600,000 atoms. Rossman's research team had to stack countless numbers of cross-sectional slices of virus crystals before they could determine the exact position of each atom.

After four years of relentless effort, the job was completed. Rossman's team produced an accurate, three-dimensional model of a rhinovirus. After centuries of battling cold viruses, humans had their first look at their ancient, unseen enemy.

It turns out that a cold virus resembles a miniature planet, complete with mountain peaks and deep canyons. Upon closer examination, researchers discovered that cold viruses are even more adept at the art of deception than was first supposed. The immune system's antibodies latch onto the "jutting mountains" in order to destroy the rhinovirus. But these protrusions come in such a fantastic array of shapes, which can vary from one generation of viruses to the next, that it's difficult for the antibodies to recognize the intruder consistently.

Scientists have also discovered how viruses are able to break into the body's cells. They found that all cells are equipped with special receptors, which they use to communicate with the rest of the body. Viruses, however, are able to use these receptors to their own advantage. They have developed a molecular structure that fits perfectly into the receptor. From that contact point, the viral nucleic acid spills into the cell.

Scientists searching for this cell-connecting structure on the virus reasoned that it should not change shape from generation to generation. If it did, it would not match up with the cell receptor. Therefore, this structure could not be in the ever-changing mountains; it must be in the canyons.

Sure enough, the cell-binding part of the virus was found to be tucked away so deep in the crevices of the canyons that even the minute antibodies are too large to reach it.

In probing for a way to neutralize the virus, there was no point in focusing on the mountains, because almost as soon as scientists could get a fix on them, they would change shape. But that constant, cell-binding portion provided a stationary target, one that could not mutate as soon as scientists had figured out how to deal with it.

Attempts to exploit this new knowledge of the rhinovirus were complicated by the fact that cells were found to have many different types of receptors. If different viruses were able to link up to different kinds of receptors, then the virus would win the numbers game again; dozens of different treatments would be necessary to block each receptor.

But further efforts by research groups uncovered a weakness in the virus's deception mechanism. It turns out that 90 percent of all rhinoviruses bond to a single type of receptor, a molecule called ICAM-1. That meant that all virologists needed to do to prevent 90 percent of colds was to foul up the virus's ability to attach to the ICAM-1.

There were two possible courses of action to prevent the virus from hooking up with the ICAM-1 receptor: 1) tie up the attaching portion of the virus so that it could not bind to the cell receptor, 2) block the receptors so that viruses could not latch onto them.

Two groups of research teams in the United States tried the first approach. They succeeded in creating a decoy ICAM-1 molecule that could lure viruses into binding with it. Any virus that attached itself to a decoy would be taken out of commission and so would be unable to link up with a real cell.

In test-tube experiments, scientists doused healthy cells with artificial ICAM-1 molecules and then introduced rhinoviruses. The decoy molecules bound up more than 90 percent of the rhinoviruses before they could infect the cells.

This suggests that it may be possible to prevent colds

by using a nasal spray containing decoy ICAM-1. The spray would soak the upper respiratory passages with these decoys, which would then sop up the viruses before they could cause a cold.

The second approach was attempted by Richard Colonno of Merck Sharp and Dohme Research Labs. Colonno believed it might be possible to custom-design a special antibody that would temporarily block the cell receptors so that the viruses could not connect with them.

Colonno's plan was to inject mice with tiny pieces of human cells that contained ICAM-1 receptors. The mouse's immune system would recognize these cells as foreign and would begin manufacturing antibodies against the receptor. Colonno could then harvest these antibodies and use them to block receptors in humans.

The mice cooperated by making antibodies against the material that Colonno injected. Unfortunately, they made thousands of kinds of antibodies, and it would be no easy matter to try and isolate which of those antibodies was custom-made to attack the ICAM-1 receptor. Colonno's team began the laborious process of locating the desired antibody. But after performing more than 8,000 experiments over eleven months without any sign that he was even on the right track, Colonno was ready to admit defeat. He decided to do one last experiment and then call it quits.

Miraculously, that last experiment came up a winner. Colonno found an antibody that not only blocked the ICAM-1 receptor, it even knocked attached rhinoviruses off the receptor.

After some further refinement of the ICAM-1 antibody, researchers were ready to give it the ultimate test. The first experiment with human volunteers ended in disaster. Despite treatment with the antibody, nearly every one of the subjects came down with a cold.

Hoping that the failure was merely a result of improper dosage, experimenters tried again using eight

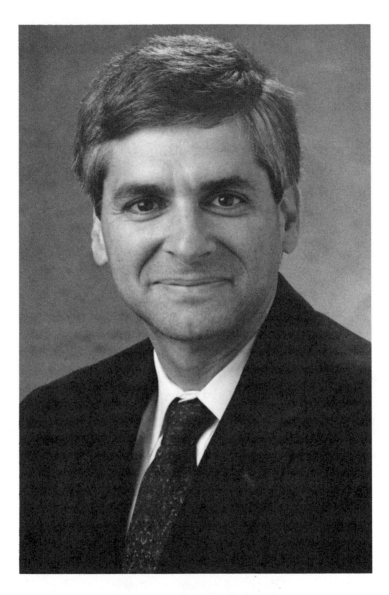

Dr. Richard Colonno is a leader in
research on receptor blockers—antibodies
that prevent cold viruses from
attaching themselves to body cells.

times the original amount of antibodies. Although the receptor blocker was soon destroyed by the immune system, it lasted long enough to delay the onset of a cold by a couple of days and to reduce the severity of the cold.

Receptor blockers, if perfected, could be used in nose drops or a nasal spray, and would be especially effective for those in close contact with others who have colds.

The technology of cell receptor blocking is still a long way from being perfected. As with all innovative research, the likelihood of side effects has yet to be determined. There is some uneasiness about tying up the cell receptors, since these are the cell's communication links. But this type of technology offers some hope, not only in fighting the relatively mild common cold but in combating more deadly viral diseases as well.

NEW DRUGS

Several chemical compounds have been shown to be effective in either preventing colds and flu or in limiting their effects.

In the mid-1950s, British researcher Alick Isaacs, with his assistant, Jean Lindenmann, added a heat-killed flu virus to chick embryo tissue. After a period of incubation, the viruses were removed, and fresh, noninfected tissue was added. This new tissue showed a strong resistance to flu viruses. The original chick cells apparently produced something that interfered with the reproduction of viruses in the second batch of healthy cells. This substance was isolated and given the name interferon.

It has since been discovered that every type of viral infection triggers the release in the body of interferon, which is manufactured by white blood cells. The substance was tested against cold infections and found to be effective in preventing colds.

If interferon were a cheap, abundant material, it could well be the answer to cold prevention. Since the substance is produced naturally by the body, it is likely to be safer than many artificially produced chemicals.

Unfortunately, cells produce only minuscule amounts of the chemical, and so for many years there was little hope of making practical use of it. However, recent advances in genetic engineering techniques have solved the problem. Certain bacteria have been programmed to produce interferon in reasonable quantities. Interferon may yet play a key role in the fight against colds and flu.

In the 1970s the drug *amantadine* was discovered to be effective in preventing flu and to reduce slightly the severity of colds. Doctors commonly recommend that those who have been exposed to type A flu begin taking amantadine immediately and continue on it for ten days. The drug provides two weeks of protection against flu, after which time a flu shot is recommended.

Research is continuing in the area of antiviral drugs. One of the main obstacles to finding an effective treatment against viral infection is finding a way to stop viruses once they penetrate a cell. Most drugs cannot remain inside the cell long enough to disarm the virus. A synthetic substance called *virazole,* created in the 1970s, could remain in the cells for as long as 12 hours. The compound, however, was found to cause birth defects in rodents, and research was discontinued.

Dr. Rossman of Purdue has been working on an alternative method of thwarting viruses. He has found a number of compounds that make the surface of a cold virus so rigid that the nucleic acid in it cannot leave the virus to take over control of the cell mechanisms.

IMMUNE SYSTEM ENABLERS

A great deal of recent research has focused on ways that people can help their immune systems perform more efficiently.

One of the areas under study is the effect of diet on

the immune system. Researchers are beginning to isolate the specific way that certain nutrients and trace elements assist the immune system:

Vitamin A, which is plentiful in carrots and yellow vegetables, is believed to stimulate antibody production.

B vitamins seem to be required for the manufacture of phagocytes. Alcohol appears to inhibit this production. Leafy green vegetables are a rich source of B vitamins.

Vitamin B6, found in whole grains, meat, and bananas, shows evidence of being involved in the formation of T cells. Mice that have been fed large amounts of vitamin B6 show a more effective immune response to infection.

Vitamin C, found in abundance in citrus fruits, may yet bear out the claims of its supporters. The vitamin may be essential in stimulating the production of interferon.

Vitamin E has been shown to protect against the effects of a hormone that causes deterioration in the immune system during the aging process.

Iron is important in building up the body's supply of white blood cells. Those with iron deficiencies have been shown to develop more upper respiratory infections than those with an adequate intake.

Zinc appears to be involved in some immune system reactions. Several years ago zinc lozenges were hailed as an effective way to reduce the severity of a cold. Recent tests have cast some doubt as to any significant benefit of zinc.

Deficiencies of any of the above elements have been shown to reduce the efficiency of the immune system. That does not mean, however, that if a little is good for you, then more must be better. Both zinc and iron, for example, can cause other health problems if taken in large amounts. But these new findings do highlight the wisdom of a healthy, sensible diet, and may provide researchers with clues as to what the body needs to ward off infection.

Researchers are also curious about the effect of exercise in warding off infection. Studies have shown that physical labor or exercise can increase the effectiveness of the immune system.

Finally, there is intense interest in the role of the mind in maintaining good health. While some medical experts caution that "it has not been shown unequivocably that someone's state of mind can cause or cure a specific disease," it has recently been demonstrated that the brain actually sends signals to and receives messages from the immune system. During times of severe stress, anxiety, grief, loneliness, and depression, the brain releases a substance called *beta endorph* that inhibits the action of certain immune cells. Relaxation studies at Harvard University found that the production of antibodies was increased in subjects who cleared their mind of all outside concerns. It may yet be discovered that good mental health is a key protection against viral infection.

None of these areas of research, from cell receptor blocks to interferon to vitamin C to mental health studies, has yet produced a cure for the common cold or flu. We cannot predict exactly where these medical advances will take us. Perhaps one day a bottle of common-cold preventative spray will be as much a part of the bathroom medicine cabinet as a bottle of aspirin. Perhaps short-term sprays will be available that people can use before a trip, when they have company, or when colds and flu are especially prevalent.

However it happens, virologists are confident that one day the common cold will not be so common, and that the flu will be a relatively rare occurrence. In the meantime, though, hang on to that box of tissues. There's more sniffling ahead for most of us.

GLOSSARY

Allergy: an extreme reaction by the immune system to relatively harmless substances, such as dust, pollen, etc.

Amantadine: a drug shown to have some value in preventing flu

Antibodies: tiny substances in the blood that latch onto and neutralize antigens

Antigens: harmful bacteria, protozoans, viruses, and toxins that invade the body

Antihistamine: drug that counteracts the effects of histamine and so relieves the symptom of runny nose in allergic reactions

Bacillus: a bacterium characterized by its rod shape

Beta endorph: substance produced by the brain during depression and stress; can reduce effectiveness of immune system

Bronchitis: infection of the bronchial tubes that lead from the trachea (throat area) to the lungs

Centrifuge: a machine that spins a chamber so rapidly that the outward (centrifugal) force causes substances with different densities to separate

Cholera: a disease that affects the digestive system

Cilia: tiny hairs that serve to clear respiratory lining of impurities

Cold: relatively mild illness caused by viral infection of upper respiratory tract

Contagious: able to pass infection easily from one person to another

Cross-reactivity: the ability of one virus to produce an immune system reaction against a different virus

Croup: viral illness, usually in small children, that causes barky cough and breathing problems

Culture: a medium specially formulated to promote growth of microorganisms in the laboratory

Epidemic: outbreak of a large number of similar infections among a local population

Flu: short for influenza; viral infection of the upper respiratory tract, similar to but more serious than common cold

Histamine: compound that is released, especially in an allergic reaction, causing runny nose

Immune system: system of substances and agents within the body that guard against infection

Immunity: protection against an illness or infection

Incubation: period during which an illness develops from initial infection into recognizable symptoms

Influenza: (see flu)

Inoculation: the transfer of an infecting agent into a healthy subject

Interferon: substance manufactured in white blood cells that interferes with viral growth

Miasma: poisonous air or atmosphere

MHC: (major histocompatibility complex)—an immune system molecule that alerts T cells to the presence of an antigen that has penetrated a body cell

Nucleic acid: master molecules (including DNA and RNA) that control the functions of cells

Pandemic: outbreak of a large number of similar infections that spreads over many countries

Phagocytes: "cell-eaters"—white blood cells that consume antigens

Placebo: medicine that contains no active ingredients, used to measure the psychological effect of a treatment as opposed to the physical effect

Pneumonia: infection or inflammation of the lungs

Replication: self-duplication or reproduction

Reye's syndrome: serious secondary illness in young children that sometimes follows type B flu

Rhinovirus: a family of viruses that makes up approximately half the known cold-causing viruses

Secondary infection: infection that occurs after an area has been weakened by an initial infection

Strep throat: illness with symptoms of sore throat and fever, caused by streptococcus bacteria

Susceptible: vulnerable or having little resistance against

Symptoms: the visible signs of an infection or disease

T cells: immune system cells programmed to recognize and attack antigens

Vaccination: treatment that brings about immunity by exposing the subject to a mild, weakened, or killed form of the disease-causing agent

Viral rhinitis: medical term for the common cold

Virazole: synthetic antiviral drug

Virologists: scientists who study viruses

Virus: submicroscopic objects that have some characteristics of living things and some characteristics of nonliving things. They consist of tiny packets of nucleic acid enclosed in protein

FOR FURTHER READING

Books

Castleman, Michael. *Cold Cures*. Columbia, New York: Fawcett, 1987.

Feltman, John, ed. *Prevention's Giant Book of Health Facts*: Emmaus, Pa., 1991.

Jensen, Marcus M. & Donald Wright. *Introduction to Medical Microbiology*. Englewood Cliffs, N.J.: Prentice-Hall, 1989.

Knight, David C. *Viruses: Life's Smallest Enemies*. New York, William Morrow, 1981.

Nourse, Alan E. *Viruses*. New York: Franklin Watts, 1983.

Pauling, Linus. *How to Live Longer and Feel Better*. New York: W.H. Freeman, 1986.

Schroeder, Steven A., ed. *Current Medical Diagnosis and Treatment 1991*. Norwalk, CT: Appleton and Lange, 1991.

Articles

Castleman, Michael. "Fast-spreading Flu; Don't Let it Catch You!" *Redbook*, January 1991.

"How to Survive a Cold." *Glamour*, February 1991.

McVeigh, Gloria. "How to Stop Your Head Cold, Cold." *Prevention*, November 1990.

Mercer, Marilyn. "The Complete Book of Colds and Flu." *Good Housekeeping*, November 1987.

Oppenheimer, Michael. "What to Do About Colds and Flu: Home Remedies Are Best." *Better Homes & Gardens*, February 1989.

Poppy, John. "Cold Comfort." *Esquire*, November 1988.

Radetsky, Peter. "Taming the Wily Rhinovirus," *Discover*, April 1989.

"Uncommon ICAM Blocks Common Cold Virus." *Science News*, March 10, 1990.

INDEX

Italicized page numbers refer to illustrations.

Adenoids, 34
Adenoviruses, *28, 29,* 30, *36*
Age and likelihood of infection, relation between, 58–59
Alcoholic beverages, 73
Allergies, 67–68
Amantadine, 83
Anthrax, 19
Antibiotics, 43
Antibodies, 35, 38, 47–48
Antigens, 35
Antihistamines, 68–69
Aspirin, 74

Bacteria, 17, 19, 22, 35
  secondary bacterial infections, 42–43
  vaccination and, 48
Beijerinck, Martinus, 21
Beta endorph, 85
Bradykinin, 68
Bronchitis, 40

Camphor, 71
Cause of colds and flu age and likelihood of:
  infection, relation between, 58–59
  air as, 15, 17, 26
  ancient beliefs about, 15
  bacteria as, 17, 19
  cold and wet conditions as, 17, 26, 55, 57
  contact with infected persons, 58–60, 63–65
  dry air and, 58
  See also Viruses
Centrifuges, 23
Chicken soup, 71
Children as carriers of viruses, 59
Cholera, 48
Cilia, 34
"Cold," origin of word, 17

Cold and wet conditions,
    17, 26, 55, 57
Colds
    allergies, similarity to,
        67–68
    attack of cold virus,
        30–41
    commonplace nature
        of, 11
    contagiousness, 11,
        59–60
    costs to society, 11
    secondary bacterial
        infections, 42–43
    symptoms, 11, 40
    vaccination and,
        53–54
    See also Cause of
        colds and flu;
        Prevention of colds
        and flu; Treatment
        of colds and flu
Cold-weather lifestyles,
    57–58
Colonno, Richard, 80, *81*
Contagiousness, 11,
    59–60
Coronaviruses, 30
Cough and sore throat
    medications, 69
Cowpox, 45, 47
Crieghton, John, 11
Cross-reactivity, 47
Croup, 41, 73

Decongestants, 69
Dick, Elliot, 32, 34
Doctor visits, 73–74

Ear infections, 41, 43
Electron microscopes, 24,
    25, 26, 31, 36
Elford, W. J., 23
Epidemics, 15
Eucalyptus, 71
Exercise, 84–85

Families, virus
    transmission in, 63–64
Flu. *See* Influenza

Genetic engineering, 83
Germ theory, 17
Gwaltny, Jack, 32

Handkerchiefs, 60
Harrison, William Henry, 17
Hendley, Owen, 32
Henson, Jim, 43
Hippocrates, 15, *16*
Histamines, 40, 68
Hong Kong flu, 41, 42
    virus, *31*
Humid air, 58, 64, 72–73

ICAM-1 molecules, 79–80
Immune system, 14
    counterattack against
        viruses, 35, *37,* 38,
        39, 40, 42
    interferon, 68,
        82–83, 84
    nutrition and, 83–84
    receptor blocking
        and, 78–80, 82
    vaccination and,
        44–45, 47–48

Influenza, 11, 14
  attack of influenza
    virus, 41–42
  contagiousness,
    59–60
  deaths from, 14
  mutation by flu virus,
    50–51
  pandemic of
    1918–19, *13,* 14,
    22, 23, 41
  seasonal occurrences,
    57–58
  secondary bacterial
    infections, 42–43
  symptoms, 40, 42
  types A, B, and C, 41
  vaccines against,
    50–51, 53
  See also Cause of
    colds and flu;
    Prevention of colds
    and flu; Treatment
    of colds and flu
"Influenza," origin of
  word, 15
Inoculation. *See*
  Vaccination
Interferon, 68, 82–83, 84
Intestinal flu, 42
Iron, 84
Isaacs, Alick, 82
Ivanoski, Dmitri, 19, 21

Jenner, Edward, 45, 47, 48

Koch, Robert, 19, *20*
Koen, J. S., 23

Laryngitis, 41
Lemon and honey
  treatment, 72
Lindenmann, Jean, 82
London flu pandemic of
  1935–36, 41

Macrophages, *37*
Measles, 22
Meister, Joseph, 49
Mental health, relation to
  physical health, 85
Menthol, 71
MHC molecule, 38
Miasma, 17
Model of cold virus, *76,*
  77, 78
Mouth's role in trans-
  mission of viruses, 60
Mucus, 34

Nasal sprays, 69
Nucleic acids, 24, 27, 50
Nutrition
  immune system and,
    83–84
  for prevention of
    colds, 61, *62,*
    83–84
  for treatment of
    colds, 73

Over-the-counter
  medications, 10, 69, *70,*
  71

Pandemics, 15

93

Pasteur, Louis, 17, *18,*
    48–49
Pauling, Linus, 61
Penicillin, 43
Pfeiffer, Richard, 19
Pfeiffer's bacillus, 19, 22
Phagocytes, 35, *37,* 38
Phipps, James, 47
Pneumonia, 40, 43
Polio, 49–50
Poverty and transmission
    of viruses, 59
Prevention of colds and
    flu, 55
        effective measures,
            63–65
        exercise and, 84–85
        humid air and, 58, 64
        mental health and, 85
        nutrition and, 61, *62,*
            83–84
        receptor blocking,
            78–80, 82
        smoking and, 61
        tissue-handkerchief
            issue, 60
        vitamin C for, 61, 63
Protozoans, 19

Rabies, 48–49
Receptor blocking, 78–80,
    82
Respiratory system, *12*
Resting the body, *56,* 67, 74
Reye's syndrome, 74
Rhinoviruses, 30
Rossman, Michael, *77,* 78,
    83

Salk, Jonas, 49
Sinusitis, 43, 67
Smallpox, 45, 47
Smoking, 61
Space shuttle, 11
Spanish flu pandemic of
    1918–19, *13,* 14, 22,
    23, 41
Stanley, Wendell, 23–24
Steam baths, 72–73
Strep throat, 74
Swine flu, 23, 51, *52*

T cells, 35, 38, *39,* 47–48
Theiler, Max, 49
Throat problems, 73–74
Tissue-handkerchief issue,
    60
Treatment of colds and
    flu, 66–67
        alcoholic beverages, 73
        antihistamines, 68–69
        chicken soup, 71
        doctor visits, 73–74
        drugs, development
            of, 82–83
        effective treatments,
            74
        future treatments, 75,
            78–80, 82–85
        humid air, 72–73
        nutrition, 73
        ointments for chest
            area, 71
        over-the-counter
            medications, 10,
            69, *70,* 71
        rest, *56,* 67, 74

Treatment of colds and flu
  (*cont.*)
    symptoms, focus on,
      67, 69
    vitamin C, 72

Vaccination, 24, *46, 52*
    bacteria and, 48
    body's response to, 51
    colds and, 53–54
    for flu virus, 50–51, 53
    origins of, 45, 47
    preparation of
      vaccines, 51
    principle behind,
      44–45, 47–48, 50
    research on, 48–50
"Vaccination," origin of
  word, 47
Vaporizers, 72–73
Viral rhinitis. *See* Colds
Virazole, 83
Virologists, 24
"Virus," origin of word, 21
Viruses, *25, 28, 29, 31, 36*
    "attack" on host cell,
      34–35, *36,* 42, 78
    body's defenses
      against, 34, 35, *37,*
      38, *39,* 40, 42
    as cause of colds and
      flu, 22, 23, 26, 30
    cell-connecting
      structure on,
      78–80, 82
    discovery of, 19, 21
    entry into body, 30,
      32, *33,* 34, 41–42

growing viruses in
  laboratories, 24
incubation period, 11,
  35, 41
"living" status, 24, 27
makeup of, 23–24,
  27, 30
model of cold virus,
  76, 77, 78
mutation by, 50–51, 54
as parasites, 30
protection against.
  See Vaccination
research on, 22–24,
  26, 32, *33,* 34,
  78–80, 82
size of, 27
spread within body,
  40–41
transmission of,
  58–60, 63–65
Vitamin A, 84
Vitamin B6, 84
Vitamin C, 10
    for prevention of
      colds, 61, 63, 84
    for treatment of
      colds, 72
Vitamin E, 84

Washington, George, 17, 66
White blood cells, 35, *37,*
  38

Yeast, 17
Yellow fever, 22, 49

Zinc, 84

ABOUT THE AUTHOR

Nathan Aaseng is the author of more than eighty nonfiction books for children and young adults. His work covers such diverse subjects as sports, inventions, zoology, and medicine. Mr. Aaseng holds a bachelor's degree in biology and English from Luther College. Before becoming a full-time writer, he worked as a microbiologist for a research firm. Nathan Aaseng resides in Eau Claire, Wisconsin, with his wife and their four children.

AFX 5950

EDUCATION